Jung's Technique of Active Imagination and Desoille's Directed Waking Dream Method

Jung's Technique of Active Imagination and Desoille's Directed Waking Dream Method brings together Carl Jung's active imagination and Robert Desoille's *"rêve éveillé dirigé*/directed waking dream" (RED) method. It studies the historical development of these approaches in Central Europe in the first half of the 20th century and explores their theoretical similarities and differences, proposing an integrated framework of clinical practice.

The book aims to study the wider European context of the 1900s which influenced the development of both Jung's and Desoille's methods. This work compares the spatial metaphors of interiority used by both Jung and Desoille to describe the traditional concept of inner psychic space in the waking dreams of Jung's active imagination and Desoille's RED. It also attempts a broader theoretical comparison between the procedural aspects of both RED and active imagination by identifying commonalities and divergences between the two approaches.

This book is a unique contribution to analytical psychology and will be of great interest for academics, researchers and post-graduate students interested in the use of imagination and mental imagery in analysis, psychotherapy and counselling. The book's historical focus will be of particular relevance to Jungian and Desoillian scholars since it is the first of its kind to trace the connections between the two schools and it gives a detailed account of Desoille's early life and his first written works.

Laner Cassar is a clinical psychologist, Jungian analyst and Gestalt psychotherapist from Malta. He holds a Ph.D. in psychoanalytic studies from the Centre of Psychoanalytic Studies at the University of Essex, UK. He is the president of the Malta Jungian Developing Group (I.A.A.P.) and the International Network for the Study of Waking Dream Therapy (I.N.S.W.D.T.).

Research in Analytical Psychology and Jungian Studies Series

Series Advisor: Andrew Samuels, Professor of Analytical Psychology, Essex University, UK

The *Research in Analytical Psychology and Jungian Studies* series features research-focused volumes involving qualitative and quantitative research, historical/archival research, theoretical developments, heuristic research, grounded theory, narrative approaches, collaborative research, practitioner-led research, and self-study. The series also includes focused works by clinical practitioners, and provides new research informed explorations of the work of C. G Jung that will appeal to researchers, academics, and scholars alike.

Books in this series:

Jungian Metaphor in Modernist Literature
Exploring individuation, alchemy and symbolism
Roula-Maria Dib

Symbolic Mental Representations in Arts and Mystical Experiences
Primordial mental activity and archetypal constellations
Giselle Manica

Jung's Technique of Active Imagination and Desoille's Directed Waking Dream Method
Bridging the Divide
Laner Cassar

The Cartesian Split
A hidden myth
Brandon Short

For more information about this series please visit: https://www.routledge.com/Research-in-Analytical-Psychology-and-Jungian-Studies/book-series/JUNGIANSTUDIES.

Jung's Technique of Active Imagination and Desoille's Directed Waking Dream Method

Bridging the Divide

Laner Cassar

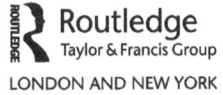
Routledge
Taylor & Francis Group

LONDON AND NEW YORK

First published 2020
by Routledge
2 Park Square, Milton Park, Abingdon, Oxon OX14 4RN

and by Routledge
605 Third Avenue, New York, NY 10017

First issued in paperback 2022

Routledge is an imprint of the Taylor & Francis Group, an informa business

Publisher's Note
The publisher has gone to great lengths to ensure the quality of this reprint but points out that some imperfections in the original copies may be apparent.

British Library Cataloguing-in-Publication Data
A catalogue record for this book is available from the British Library

Library of Congress Cataloging-in-Publication Data
A catalog record has been requested for this book

ISBN: 978-0-367-51862-2 (pbk)
ISBN: 978-1-138-31870-0 (hbk)
ISBN: 978-0-429-45439-4 (ebk)

DOI: 10.4324/9780429454394

Typeset in Sabon
by codeMantra

For my parents
 Joseph and Violet
 With gratitude

Contents

Figures

Figures

Foreword by Christian Gaillard

Emergence, regression and thinking

Very often at the heart of our relationships with ourselves, with others and with the world, we find ourselves struck by unpredicted and unpredictable events. These experiences can be sometimes serendipitous, occasionally disturbing and often quite enigmatic.

One possible reaction to these happenings is to either deny that something has emerged or else ignore them. We close the door, remaining defensive. Moreover, we find ourselves betting on our ability to avoid or outwit our malevolent encounters, the hazardous and confusing byways that may attract us and the adventures that may befall us, off the beaten path.

Robert Desoille and Carl Gustav Jung both had a taste for discovery, exploration, and bold and daring thinking, each in his own way. Both of them also enjoyed meeting other people. Yet it so happens that they barely knew each other, communicating with each other only from afar.

The author of this book brings Desoille and Jung together, which is unusual. In doing so, he creates and maps a field where these two clinicians and thinkers converse, and offers us possibilities how we might continue to further build on their ideas.

This book is both retrospective and prospective. It is retrospective in that it explores and evaluates the approaches of these two researchers, both of whom sought ways to mobilise the imagination and activate its transformative powers.

Desoille and Jung moved forward in different ways, but they have one crucial thing in common: each was careful to make room for the happy or disturbing strangeness of what is presented and represented in our relationships to ourselves; to recognise these occurrences, in their entirety and also to observe the way these occurrences resist what we wish to do with and think of them.

Hence the originality of each man's clinical practice. Their thinking was asserted independently, unintimidated and unswayed by prevailing trends. Both Desoille and Jung ventured well beyond the outlines of established psychologies.

One of this book's qualities is to show this clearly. It also sheds light on how these two researchers stood out, in their time, as theorists of emergence, long before the recognition of emergentism today. Over the past few decades, and especially the past several years, emergentism has been established as a fruitful approach in social science, biology, neurosciences and, of course, psychoanalysis.

The forward-looking dimension of their approaches develops from this focus. They trusted in the ability of the psyche to express itself. They were confident that the creativity of the soul is often a source of becoming.

Robert Desoille and Carl Gustav Jung accompanied their patients, wondering where and how far they would go, keeping them safe from threats and traps. Both of them thought and worked, more or less explicitly, in terms of processes. Accompanying the patient's journey, they were open to perspectives that sometimes suddenly appear along the way, requiring that the patient take a position, and commit.

Both Desoille and Jung had a sense of and an appreciation for the symbolic life. Hence, their attentiveness to the vivid and picturesque expressions, often structured as dramas, that may unfold in dreams or waking fantasies, when one learns how to make room for, accompanies and supports them.

They were both open to states and movements of regression. In contrast to the clarity and determination of our deliberate attitudes, intentions and plans, these regressive states bring out emotions etched in the body, and usually relegated to the margins of our daily lives.

Robert Desoille invited his patients to lie on a couch and relax by practising Schultz's autogenic training. Today, some of the clinicians inspired by Desoille's work follow the same guidelines. The patient, letting his or her body take and find its place, feels what then happens, all the way down to the deepest inner pulsations. Time is slowed down and judgement is suspended. This state of body-mind fosters a very peculiar attentiveness to oneself, and to what might then emerge.

Jung offered his patients a chair rather than a couch. Today, many of us do invite patients to lie down. But Jung knew how to demonstrate a keen presence, an emotional and physical involvement in his patients' analyses. He had learned how to give form to the sensations and transformations dwelling within the person. He himself had experienced it as a child, when he was playing at building little houses and villages with pieces of wood and stones found on the bank of the Lake Zurich. As an adult, he made stone and wood sculptures, and spent many years on the calligraphic script and paintings of his *Red Book*.

Yet Jung and Desoille had strikingly different relationships to time and history. Robert Desoille practised intense, intensive, active psychotherapies. He assigned himself the role of guide to his patients like a mountain guide. He could lead his patients, giving them instructions, while being careful to assure and reassure them through the difficult passages in their "waking dreams." His goal was to achieve observable success with his therapies, in a limited amount of time, if possible.

Unlike Desoille, Jung invited his patients to find their own pace and to create their own means of expression. He sought to accompany rather than guide them through a clinical work of transformation. It could take a long time. Following him, today, the work usually takes even longer.

For Jung, and since Jung, the point of this transformation is an individuation process that may take a lifetime, and even proves to be transgenerational as well. It belongs to a history coming from the remote past – the history of a heritage to be brought to life, experienced and renewed in the present.

As for the two men's ways of thinking, they diverge. This book shows Desoille proceeding by successively formulating several types of hypotheses. Jung's thinking also evolved, and transformed itself from one period of his life and work to another. But it adopted a form and dynamic that lasted throughout his life, by giving rise to lively, vivid, almost personified and even gendered concepts, like the *shadow*, *anima*, *animus* and the *self*, in particular. This never fails to surprise and provoke epistemologists, even today.

It remains that the two men are cousins in that both were constantly concerned with calling us to our responsibility in what shall become of a world that is trying to reinvent itself.

One of the virtues of this book, and its strength, is to point out the similarities between these two thinkers, and to open the way to a clinical practice that bridges their approaches according to current clinical theoretical developments.

Christian Gaillard

Doctor of psychology – Psychoanalyst

Former president of the S.F.P.A. and I.A.A.P.

Former professor at the National Academy of Fine Arts, Paris

Translated from French by Anita Conrade

Preface and acknowledgements

This book is based on a Ph.D. thesis completed at the Centre for Psycho-analytic Studies, University of Essex. In my Ph.D., I wanted to research the imagination in analytical psychology. However, the emphasis on originality led me to explore the work of a lesser known figure in psychology, namely Robert Desoille, and to possibly compare his work to that of Carl Jung. Little did I know that I would devote eight years researching Jung's technique of active imagination and Robert Desoille's directed waking dream and that I would discover their correspondence.

I would like to take this opportunity to show my gratitude towards several people and institutions that were instrumental in the realisation of this project. First of all, I would like to thank my supervisor Prof. Andrew Samuels for his wise counsel and encouragement to complete this thesis as well as the two board supervisors namely Prof. Renos Papadoupolos and Ms. Sue Kegerreis who provided the necessary tension for my creativity to unfold.

In particular, my deep gratitude goes to Mr. Andreas Jung, Jung's grandson, who was kind enough to welcome me in C.G. Jung's house and who helped identify Desoille's book in Jung's personal library in Zurich. I am also very much indebted to Dr. Voegli of the "E.T.H. library" in Zurich, who helped me find my way through C.G. Jung's correspondence over the years. I would also like to thank the "(C) Foundation of the Works of C. G. Jung, Zurich" that granted me permission to publish the letter Jung's secretary sent to Desoille.

I would also like to thank Dott. Alberto Passerini of S.I.S.P.I., Italy, who was instrumental towards a more in-depth understanding of Desoille's theory, and who put me in contact with the psychoanalyst M. Nicole Fabre, a patient of Desoille himself. I am also indebted to my friend Dr. Philippe Grosbois who gave me so much material published and unpublished on Andre Virel and the S.I.T.I.M. school of Oneirotherapy and to Dr. Hector Anastasia from S.U.E.D., Uruguay who helped me extend my research on the waking dream in South America.

Since I cannot mention everyone who helped me in the completion of this project, I would like to show my appreciation to the following institutions: S.I.S.P.I., G.I.R.E.P., S.U.E.D., S.A.S.D.A.D., the Picture Archives of the C.G. Jung Institute, Zurich, and the Psychology Club Zurich, the library of the University of Malta, University of Turin, *Bibliotheque Nationale de Paris, Bibliotheque National de Geneve, Institut Charles Baudouin, Institut Metapsychique International*, the *Bibliotheque d'Histoire de la Medicine et d'Ethique Medicale*, the *Bibliotheque de la Sorbonne, Association l'Elan Retrouve*, Forum 104 (Rue de Vaugirard Paris), *le Service d'État Civil de la Ville de Paris, Marie de Pellouailles le Vignes, Amis de Gilbert Marcel, Municipale de Besancon, Archives de Jean Jacques Rousseau, Association des amis de Gaston Bachelard, Association amis de Gilbert Durand, Collection de l'Art Brut, Lausanne, Institut Francaise de Psychosyntese*, the *Istituto di Psicosintesi, Société d'Etudes du Psychodrame Pratique et Théorique*, and the American Institute of Mental Imagery.

Most importantly, I could not have given this work the passion and commitment I did without the love and the patience of my family and friends. Finally, I express my deepest gratitude to the spirit and memory of Jung and Desoille for their invaluable contribution to the study of the imagination in psychotherapy.

Introduction

This book presents a rapprochement between two psychotherapeutic methods that rely on the use of the imagination, i.e., C.G. Jung's active imagination technique and Robert Desoille's *"rêve éveillé dirigé*/directed waking dream" (RED) method. Both active imagination and directed waking dream therapy are similar yet distinct methods, used to access the unconscious, which developed in different places in the early decades of the twentieth century. These two methods were eventually utilised for psychotherapeutic purposes.

This book strives to enrich C.G. Jung's analytical psychology with Desoille's psychotherapeutic method of *rêve éveillé dirigé* and the imaginative psychotherapeutic methods of post-Desoillian thinkers. For a long time, Jungian active imagination has distanced itself from the French method. As such, a relationship between the two was deemed almost impossible, after being judged so by Jung's close and influential disciple, the Jungian analyst Marie L. von Franz (1980). To the contrary, French post-Freudians seem to have embraced the *rêve éveillé dirigé* method and given it a Freudian or Lacanian dimension (Launay, Levine & Maurey, 1975; Dufour, 1978; Fabre, 1979; Fabre & Maurey, 1985; Maurey, 1995).

This book questions the main arguments raised by some Jungians who were ambivalent towards the *rêve éveillé dirigé* approach and investigates historical incidents that have led to such an outcome. It also highlights the moments when Jungians co-operated with Desoillians. Since post-Jungians have developed the classical idea of active imagination, the time is ripe to attempt to re-open a possible dialogue between these two approaches which initially occurred in the first half of the twentieth century and has remained blocked ever since. It also follows the quite recent publication of Jung's (2009) *Liber Novus – The Red Book*, which has led to renewed interest on active imagination, amongst academics as well as practitioners (Ashton, 2010; Schwartz-Salant, 2010; Ulanov, 2010; Brutsche, 2011; Bishop, 2012; Drob, 2012; Gaillard, 2012; Shamdasani, 2012; Stein, 2012; Rowland, 2013; Connolly, 2014; Kirsch & Hogenson, 2014).

Active imagination

The technique of active imagination was developed by the Swiss psychiatrist and psychoanalyst Carl Jung (1875–1961) between 1913 and 1916 to work with one's imagination. Jung's understanding of active imagination developed over time. He uses the term "active imagination" for the first time in the *Tavistock Lectures* in 1935. Before this date Jung referred to his therapeutic method with different names such as the "transcendent function," "active fantasy," "visioning," "dialectical method," "technique of introversion" and "introspection." Jung's active imagination moves from a technique to a central method of how to practise analytical psychology. Jung's first major paper on this technique is *The Transcendent Function* (1916/1960), which he originally wrote in 1916 and later revised, before it was included in his *Collected Works*. Despite some changes in the content of the original script, namely "the greater centrality of the opposites, the increased emphasis on meaning and purpose, and the creation of a living third thing" (Miller, 2004, p. 30), the core concepts about his method of engaging with the unconscious remained untouched. In his final opus, *Mysterium Coniunctionis*, Jung (1955/1970) described active imagination as the way towards self-knowledge and individuation.

Carl Jung developed this technique as one of several that would define his distinctive contribution to the practice of psychotherapy. In a letter of February 15, 1955 to A. M. Hubbard, he describes active imagination as an example of an "analytical method of psychotherapy" (Jung, 1975, p. 222). Jung's paper, *The Transcendent Function*, outlines the procedure for practising active imagination, although he further elaborated it in later works and personal correspondences as we will see in the next chapter. Jung included the term "active imagination" retrospectively when he added a prefatory note to his essay.

Active imagination is a method for tapping into one's unconscious. In active imagination, there is an active weakening of normal daytime consciousness, a Janetian *"abaissement du niveau mental*/reduction in mental level," in order to focus on the inner world. The person doing it may choose to focus on a constellation of unconscious material such as a feeling, an obsessive thought, a dream scene or an image to which one feels drawn. It is important to exert as little influence as possible on mental images as they unfold. Jung referred to this meditative part in terms of *wu wei*, that is, the Taoist idea of letting things happen (Jung, 1931/1967, p. 16 [CW13, para. 20]). In one of the *Visions Seminars* of May 4, 1932, he explained how he used to encourage practitioners of this method to observe the scene in a special attentive way referred to as *betrachten* (Jung, 1998, p. 661) until things move spontaneously, and report them, rather than to consciously fill the scene with one's desired changes. He would then encourage them to step into the images and if it is a speaking one, to engage in dialogue with it so as to communicate with the figure and to listen to what he or she has to say back.

Jung always allowed freedom for the images to speak for themselves. After this interaction between the unconscious and the conscious mind, the patient can write or draw what he or she has experienced (Dallett, 1982). After the affects and images of the unconscious have flown into awareness, the ego actively enters into the experience. Any arising insights must be converted into an ethical obligation, i.e., to live it in life. Jung referred to this part as *auseinandersetzung*, which is usually translated as a confrontation or a "coming to terms with the Other in us" (Jung, 1955/1970, [CW14, para. 706]), i.e., with the unconscious.

In active imagination, unlike daydreaming, the ego takes responsibility in the same manner that it would if the imaginal sequence were an actual waking situation. Jung differentiated between passive activity with unconscious fantasies that were "involuntary" and occurred when one "was lost in his dreams" (Jung, 1913/1970, p. 185 [CW4, para. 417]) and "active" or waking fantasy activity that occurred when one "deliberately turned his attention to his inner life [....] he must now think, consciously and intentionally" (ibid., p. 186). As a result, active imagination engages complexes rather than using the imaginal ability as in daydreaming to escape from such conflict.

Jung suggested that active imagination should be done when one is alone after an analysis has ended or when the patient's ego is strong enough to face the contents of the unconscious. He believed that since it is performed when one is alone, patients have less transference complications and the patient is not subjected to the therapist's influence. Active imagination can also be done through visualisation, automatic writing, or by artistic activities such as dance, music, painting, sculpting or playing with sand.

Rêve Eveillé Dirigé (RED). Another imaginative therapy created by Robert Desoille in the early 1920s, which is based on waking dreams, is the "*rêve éveillé dirigé*/directed waking dream" method. The directed waking dream is somewhat like conscious dreaming in that we are able to communicate with aspects of our inner self. For Desoille (1966), it is a method of exploring, understanding and even transforming, through imagery, the inexhaustible reservoir of accumulated anxieties, fears, desires and hopes.

In this method, a person stretches out on a couch and becomes comfortably relaxed. Then, with the help of a guide or therapist, he or she is given an initial image as a stimulus to focus on. He or she is then encouraged to enter, ascend or descend in imagery and report the images that are encountered while verbalising to the therapist what he or she is experiencing. Through the method of ascending in imaginative space, a person comes into contact with his or her higher potentialities and spiritual tendencies, while descending brings the patient in contact with his or her instincts and primitive drives (Desoille, 1938).

There are several ways in which the therapist can direct the patient's daydream session such as reminding him or her that in a waking dream anything can happen, encouraging the patient to explore the heights or depths of the imaginative space and intervening when the imagery gets too threatening so as to prevent intense anxiety. In another phase of the therapeutic work, the subject writes a report of his waking dream experience which will then be used in a face-to-face session in order to explore the meaning of the scenario.

The *rêve éveillé dirigé* is a similar yet distinct imaginative technique to active imagination, thus making it conducive to comparison. Between the two approaches there is a tension between their respective use of undirected and directed imagination. RED is less directive than it seems at face value, while there is an element of directivity in active imagination even though it comes across as a non-directive technique. A critique of the two approaches is important for several reasons. First of all, this book aims to provide a robust and more comprehensive theoretical comparison of RED with active imagination. It explores the basic epistemological assumptions behind both approaches and their compatibility. This is done first by evaluating the arguments brought forward by classical Jungians against the possible integration of the directed waking dream method with active imagination and then by questioning the conclusions reached. Furthermore, it also explores the "why" and the "when," and more importantly the "how," RED can be introduced in the analytic session and integrated with active imagination. This critical comparison finally leads us to the development of a framework of a RED-based approach to active imagination. Such a comparison provides an academic background presented as a hybridised integration of the practice of the directed waking dream method in the analytical session. This book is primarily aimed for those analytical psychologists known as "medial practitioners" (Samuels, 1985), who identify neither as classical/ symbolic nor developmental/dialectic analysts. This work can provide them with another method of how to use the classical technique of active imagination in therapy. The comparison can also prove to be of benefit to the Jungian expressive arts which can make better use of the visualisation modality as part of their practice.

Since both active imagination and RED have remained rather marginal in psychotherapy, one can object to the proposal of a framework made out of these lesser known approaches which can arguably be weaker than the original approaches. However, I believe that the integration of RED with active imagination can help to make active imagination more accessible to analysts and their patients, and can help re-awaken interest in this technique. It can also give practitioners a theoretical compass of how to navigate, while in therapy, rather than resort to ad hoc procedures when it comes to using visualisation in the analytic session. RED practitioners can also benefit by deepening their method with insights arising from Jungian and post-Jungian teachings.

In this work, the less-known (in the English-speaking world) French *rêve éveillé dirigé* method serves as the other, as well as the shadow of the active imagination technique. I strive to maintain both poles of the comparative relationship – the more familiar active imagination and the less known and foreign, *rêve éveillé dirigé* – in order to bring out both the similarities and divergences between the two approaches. *Rêve éveillé dirigé* serves as an initial stimulus for active imagination itself so as to enable it to engage in a self-reflexive process. Qualities such as therapist's guidance vs. auto-guidance, directiveness vs. spontaneity, movement of image vs. staying long with one image, relaxation and body grounding vs. absence of relaxation, brief vs. long-term work and by-passing vs. working through resistance challenge us to look at active imagination differently. This exercise will allow active imagination to reclaim and integrate certain disowned and split-off aspects.

The theoretical comparison is presented as part of a broader historical investigation of the historical correspondence and references between Jung and Desoille, as well as between Jung and Desoille's disciples in the twentieth century. The lack of historical coverage on the two imaginative approaches in question is also one of the many examples in the history of psychotherapy which is full of historical gaps, unbalanced views and inexactness. Major celebratory histories of psychology have differentiated, in the words of Nicholas Rose (1996), the "sanctioned" from the "lapsed." Psychology's history can benefit from a reflexive evaluative assessment. The first part of this inquiry will focus on the "lapsed."

Thus, this work is of interest for scholars engaged in the history of psychotherapy since it focuses around the parallel development of RED with active imagination in the first part of the twentieth century. In particular, it focuses on the specific history of the debate amongst Jungian analysts on directing waking dreams, as well as instances of their collaboration with directed waking dream therapists. It also highlights the discrepancy between what Jung theorised on active imagination and his actual practice of active imagination which has generated misunderstanding amongst Jungians. In the following chapters, we will see how post-Jungians (Davidson, 1966; Garufi, 1977; Plateo-Zoja, 1978; Humbert, 1980; Samuels, 1985; Schaverien, 2007) have tried to address this inconsistency in different ways. The historical account unfolds in Europe with Switzerland as its axis, shifting west towards France and England, east towards Austria and Hungary, north towards Germany and south towards Italy.

The Swiss city of Geneva, which kept a neutral stance in terms of affinities of psychoanalytic schools, plays a key role in the historical connections between Jung and Desoille. The Genevan psychoanalyst Charles Baudouin (1893–1963) acts as a bridge between Jung and Desoille and Jungians and Desoillians. The Swiss were not prejudiced against the Germans as opposed to the French (Cifali, 1995). In France of the 1900s, there was a pervasive anti-German sentiment and reactionary nationalism which coloured the milieu of the *Belle Époque* and the early interwar years. During this period, several French names dominated the scene in experimental and clinical psychology, namely Charcot, Bernheim, Ribot, Binet, Janet and Bergson (Ellenberger, 1970). Freud was heavily resisted by his French rival Pierre Janet, and the French were still dominated by a Cartesian philosophy which left very little space for the unconscious.[1] Two of the most important critics of Freud in France were Politzer (1928/1994) and Dalbiez (1936/1941). As a result, psychoanalysis came to be seen as a Teutonic invention aimed primarily at cultural domination (Roudinesco, 1982). It was much later, after the Second World War, that the French became open to receiving ideas from American psychoanalysts (de Mijolla, 2012) and could finally embrace psychoanalysis.

Yet even when Freud became well known in France, Jung remained a marginal figure despite the small group formed in 1928 by Jean Bruneton in Paris called "Le club Gros Caillou." Jung's alleged connections to the Nazis during the Second World War did not help him become accepted by the French (Kirsch, 2000, p. 156). Moreover, in his books Jung gave very little acknowledgement to French sources and as a result he was more resisted than Freud in France. In his major works Jung paid less homage to great French thinkers such as Descartes (Kemp, 1950) but did reference Janet, Bergson, Levy-Bruhl and Binet. Jung chose to mention more French popular writers such as Anatole France, Paul Bourget, Alphonse Daudet and Pierre Benoît (David, 1973). Furthermore, Jung's lack of popularity in France was worsened by the unchronological order in which Jung's works were translated (with Jung's approval) into French. The early translations were also found to be inexact. Two of the first translators of Jung's work were the translations of the Genevan Yves Le Lay and the German doctor Roland Cahen Salebelle[2] (David, 1973).

Despite the early French reluctance to engage with Freud's ideas, Desoille took several ideas from Freud, such as the idea of repression and sublimation. He also did not shy away from integrating Jung's ideas into his work. Desoille deepened his work on the waking dream method through Jung's ideas of the collective unconscious which were included in one of his books *"Le Rêve éveillé en Psychothérapie: Essai sur la Fonction de Régulation de l'Inconscient Collectif*/The Waking Dream in Psychotherapy: Essay on the Regulatory Function of the Collective Unconscious," published in 1945.

A historical retrospective analysis

In line with Furumoto's view of history (1989), this book attends to the context and more specifically to the geographical and therapeutic contexts surrounding the two figures under investigation. I develop my historical account by relying on primary sources and archival material, and the knowledge of pertinent secondary sources so as to avoid *interprefaction*, i.e., "the manner in which interpretations and constructions are treated as facts" (Shamdasani, 2005, p. 4). The primary works on active imagination and those of the *rêve éveillé dirigé* method will serve as the *prima materia* of this comparative work between the two approaches. Moreover, secondary sources from the works of Jung and Desoille's disciples and post-Jungian and post-Desoillian writers will also be perused. Another important source of information is Jung and Desoille's analysands' testimonials, or diaries of imaginal dialogues of their waking dreams such as those of Christiana Morgan, Tina Keller, Anna Marjula, Marie-Clotilde and Juliet Favez-Boutonnier.

I rely on English, Italian, French and South American literature on the waking dream subject, most times in the original language. Some of Desoille's French work has started to be translated into English[3] only recently, although some of his work and that of his followers has been translated into Italian. As a result, I will be using the works in the original languages adding my own translation.

The historical part of this book builds upon the tradition of some academics who have also considered the relationship between analytical psychology and history. The most noteworthy contributors are Shamdasani (2003/2004), Clarke (1992, 1994) and Lu (2011, 2012). I intend to show preference for historicism over presentism, discontinuity over continuity and reflection and critique over celebration. Nonetheless, even though the historical account slouches more towards an approach of historicism rather than presentism, I see it more as an account of "presentist historicism" (Teo, 2005). This is because the interest in this research has emerged from the present state of therapeutic imagery in analytical psychology. I propose a practice framework of how active imagination can be updated with RED, after theoretically comparing the two approaches.

A comparative framework

The final section of the book will feature a comparative methodology. Comparison is inherent in all science, including social ones, where comparative research has historically played a significant role in their development as scientific disciplines (Smelser, 1976; Øyen, 1990; Ragin, 1991). Lijphart (1971) situated the comparative method as a basic method in its own right, alongside the experimental, statistical and case study methods. This work compares the spatial metaphors of interiority used by both Jung and Desoille to describe the traditional concept of inner psychic space in the waking dreams of active imagination and RED. It also attempts a broader theoretical comparison between the procedural aspects of both RED and active imagination by identifying commonalities and divergences between the two approaches. Such a comparison also helps to explore the implications of a hybridised and integrated framework for the clinical practice of a RED-based approach to active imagination. The latter fills an important gap in post-Jungian writings on active visual imagination, as well as offering a long-awaited acknowledgement of the RED method.

I hope that as the reader "tours" through space and time, science and philosophy, psychoanalysis and experimental psychology, parapsychology and spiritualism, literature and art, he or she will get a better picture of their input in the therapeutic practice of the imagination. Most importantly, I wish the reader can continue to appreciate Jung's useful technique of active imagination as it is enriched with the directed waking dream of Desoille and introduced as an integral part of analysis.

**

The structure of the book consists of three parts. Part I presents a description of the technique of active imagination and the directed waking dream method. It focuses on post-Jungian and post-Desoillian developments of both methodologies. It also describes the different arguments brought forward by Jungians in favour and against the directed waking dream.

Chapter 1 focuses on the technique of active imagination. It gives a detailed account of the circumstances which led Jung to develop this technique. It also explores the "why," "when," "what," "where" and "how" of this technique. Finally, it focuses on why Jung kept a low profile on this method.

Chapter 2 describes the development of the directed waking dream method from esoteric purposes to psychotherapeutic ones. It describes the procedures of the method and how it evolved as an alternative to psychoanalysis. It also traces the theoretical influences of Janet, Freud, Jung and finally Pavlov on Desoille's directed waking dream.

Chapter 3 focuses on the post-Jungian developments on the technique of active imagination. It also considers the role given to active imagination in different Jungian schools and how analysis can be seen as a form of active imagination. Finally, it describes how active imagination has been applied to various other disciplines and compared to other methods.

Chapter 4 deals with the main different developments of the directed waking dream after Desoille's death in the humanistic, transpersonal and psychoanalytic schools. It also describes how Desoille's legacy can still be found in different parts of the world.

Chapter 5 looks at what several Jungians had to say about the directed waking dream, some clearly dissociating themselves from the directive element of the waking dream while others remaining more inclusive and in favour of the method.

Part II is a historical investigation of the correspondence and references between Jung and Desoille, as well as between Jung and Desoille's disciples in the twentieth century.

Chapter 6 looks at the various common sources of theoretical influences in the work of Jung and Desoille including spirtistic, occult practice, as well as psychical and metapsychical research. It also considers the influence of Pierre Janet and Henri Bergson on Jung and Desoille.

Chapter 7 traces the several common teachers, friends and acquaintances that Jung and Desoille shared given the proximity of Switzerland to France.

Chapter 8 brings to light Desoille's effort to correspond with Jung. It also highlights other different practitioners who similarly tried to communicate with Jung regarding their different therapeutic methods of using the imagination.

Chapter 9 investigates the various Jungians who collaborated with Desoillians and who actively bridged differences between the two approaches.

Part III is devoted to comparing active imagination with the directed waking dream. It starts by exploring the roots of the notion of interiority in psychology and moves to an analysis of the different spatial metaphors of interiority in Jung's and Desoille's methods. This is followed by a critical theoretical comparison between the active imagination and the directed waking dream which leads to a proposed RED-based approach to active imagination.

Chapter 10 explores the notion of interiority from antiquity to modern times from a philosophical, spiritual and literary perspective. It also throws light on how these notions have influenced and permeated the work of Jung and Desoille.

Chapter 11 analyses the spatial metaphors on interiority in Jung's active imagination and Desoille's directed waking dream method. While Jung insists on facing the depths in one's unconscious, Desoille has a preference for the heights.

Chapter 12 focuses on the comparative methodology of comparing theoretically the two therapeutic approaches. The methodology is built on an assimilative integration model. This ensures that the theoretical comparison will help to identify commonalities as well as divergences between RED and active imagination and will lead to an integrated-hybrid model of a RED-based approach to active imagination named Imaginative Movement Therapy (I.M.T.).

Chapter 13 compares the two approaches from the point of view of the first two categories namely: setting and preparation of the body, and structure and directivity by the therapist. These two categories have to do with the initial stages of the therapeutic process.

Chapter 14 deals with three concepts, namely transferential and countertransferential relationship, narratives and interpretation, which will help to complete the theoretical comparison. These categories are more related to the middle and final phase of psychotherapy treatment.

I end with a conclusion which brings together the whole work.

Notes

1 Freud's early ideas were promoted in France by a small group of people in the medical field, named the *Evolution Psychiatrique* group, which included Hesnard, Régis, Allendy and Edouard Pichon (David, 1973). They were also in contact during the inter-war period with a group of French-speaking Swiss psychoanalysts from Geneva who also helped to keep psychoanalysis alive in France. These included the psychologist Thoedore Flournoy; the psychiatrist Edouard Claparede; the psychoanalysts Charles Odier, Charles Baudouin and Raymond de Saussure most of whom were related to each other by blood (Cifali, 1995). Baudouin himself did not adhere to orthodox Freudianism and turned to Carl Jung and Alfred Adler for the theoretical elements that he felt were relevant to clinical work. Baudouin gave space to Desoille to publish his waking dream method in one of his journals (Desoille, 1938).

2 Roland Cahen Salabelle also met Desoille and had tried three or four waking dream therapy sessions with Desoille himself. This is written in part of a correspondence Desoille had with his friend the Swiss educator Adolph Ferriere between 1936 and 1949 found in the archives of the *Institut Jean Jacques Rousseau* in Geneva – Fonds A. Ferrière, dossier AdF/C/1/18. Cahen Salabelle was analysed by Jung himself and was crucial to the development of analytical psychology after the Second World War with the founding of the *Société C. G. Jung* in 1954. He also arranged the meeting of Jung with Lacan (Kirsh, 2000, pp. 157–158).

3 The Inner Garden Foundation through Inner Garden Press has so far translated three books of Desoille.

Part I

Active imagination and the directed waking dream

Chapter 1

Active imagination

Jung's interest in the imaginal arose from his maternal side of the family who were into spiritualism, especially his mother. As a child, Jung sensed that he was in fact two different persons, called "Personality No. 1" (the young boy growing up in Klein Huningen near Basle) and "Personality No. 2" (the eternal and timeless side of himself, his own "other"). Moreover, in his childhood, Jung experienced several visual hallucinations. He appeared to have had the ability to evoke fantasies voluntarily. However, Jung in his youth did not always give so much weight to images as he did to the mental faculties of abstract thinking deeming them "thoroughly immoral from an intellectual viewpoint" (Jung, 1925/1989, p. 27). His conversion to holding images in positive regard had been so drastic that in his late life he attributed his creative work to the fantasies which he had in 1912: "Everything that I accomplished in later life was already contained in them, although at first only in the form of emotions and images" (Jung, 1963/1995, p. 217).

After his break-up with Freud in 1912, Jung went through "a period of inner uncertainty [...] a state of disorientation" (Jung, 1963/1995, p. 194). Although Jung had established himself professionally in his psychiatric career as well as in the psychoanalytic movement of his time, he felt that he had lost his soul. This was a time of intense personal analysis for Jung. Jung put himself as the object of the experiment, while the unconscious is the subject carrying out the experiment (ibid., p. 202). Jung retreated to his study and allowed his mind to wander far in both fantasies and waking dreams unrestrained by convention, reason or conscious control.

Jung (2009) described his confrontations with his unconscious in *The Red Book*. This phase lasted more than four years, and he found himself again and again in danger of being overwhelmed by the unconscious and its numinous contents. Jung was not content with the contemplation of his visions; he followed up his reflections with a rational integration of his observations and experiences. Jung wrote down and drew his imaginary dialogues, dream explorations, pictures and thoughts, in notebooks which later became known as *The Red Book*. He wrote them down in a style similar to St. Augustine's *Confessions* and Nietzche's *Zarathusra*.

In *The Red Book*, Jung slowly acknowledged the other within him. Jung's psyche chooses Elijah and Salome amongst others as personifications of his unconscious thoughts. Some of the fantastical figures are human, while others were divine or mythical. In *Liber Primus*, he met these figures accompanied by a guide while he is unattended in the *Liber Secundus*. These figures helped Jung look at and reflect on his own ugly side, his overdeveloped rationality and his underdeveloped feeling function. Jung engaged with these images by forming a dialogue with them. In these dialogues a common feature is the asking of the names of these imaginative figures. Jung met them with respect and did not revere them as gods, because they were not. He questioned them and challenged them. Furthermore, Jung did not identify with them and kept a distance from them.

As a result of this experience with interior images from his unconscious, Jung developed a waking dream technique which he later named "active imagination." Gradually, he started recommending this practice to his analysands (Douglas, 1993; Swan 2007).

Fantasy thinking: the precursor of active imagination

Jung did not refer to his method as active imagination from the beginning of his writings or lectures. Jung used the term "active imagination" for the first time in public during the question time following the last of his lectures in London at the Tavistock Clinic in autumn of 1935. The lecture notes were circulated privately in mimeograph in 1936 but were not published during Jung's life (Merkur, 1993).

Jung's writings about his method of active imagination were preceded by many references to *fantasy thinking* of which he contrasts with *directed thinking*. For Jung, the former is like Freud's primary process thinking, while the latter can be compared to Freud's secondary process thinking. In *Symbols of Transformation*, Jung describes *directed thinking* as deliberate, organised and purposeful whilst *fantasy thinking* as spontaneous, associative and directionless. Fantasy thinking leads away from reality into fantasies of the past or future. By contrast, *directed thinking* turns outwards to the world and, like Freud, it operates through the reality principle. However, Jung differs from Freud on the notion of *fantasy thinking*. Freud argued that *fantasy thinking* operates by the pleasure principle, i.e., that fantasy is a wish-fulfilling activity that can arise when an instinctual wish is frustrated (Freud, 1908/1972, pp. 34–43). In *The Structure of the Unconscious*, Jung challenges the Freudian and Adlerian meaning of fantasy as a symbolic disguise for basic drives and describes it as:

> the creative matrix of everything that has made progress possible for humanity. Fantasy [...] is a psychic function that has its roots in the

conscious and the unconscious alike, in the individual as much as in the collective.

(Jung, 1916/1966, p. 290 [CW7, para. 490])

From phantasia to imagination

In *Psychological Types*, Jung deepens his reflections on *fantasy thinking* by differentiating two types of *fantasy thinking*, namely "passive fantasy" and "active fantasy" (Jung, 1921/1971, p. 428 [CW6, para. 712]). Passive fantasy is a subjective figment of the mind whilst active fantasy is an image-making, form-creative activity. In his distinction of terms, he seemed to have been following the medieval alchemists who emphasised the difference between daydreams and creative imagination or *phantasia* and *imaginatio*. In fact, in *The Tavistock Lectures* he equated "active fantasy" with imagination proper "per veram imaginationem et non phantastica" and explained that fantasy is "mere nonsense" while imagination is "active purposeful creation" (Jung, 1935/1976, p. 171 [CW18, para. 396]). He further maintained that whereas "active fantasy" is "evoked by an attitude directed to the perception of unconscious contents, as a result of which the libido immediately invests all of the elements emerging from the unconscious," in the case of "passive fantasy," this does not occur (Jung, 1921/1971, p. 428 [CW6, para. 712]).

Fantasy: from the realms of infancy and mental illness to the dead

Jung did not relegate unconscious fantasies to an infantile imaginative activity although they are "apparently infantile reminiscences [...] they are not themselves infantile" (Jung, 1912/1967, pp. 28–29 [CW5, para. 38]). Yet, fantasies allow man to be playful and in *Psychological Types*, he stated that the "dynamic principle of fantasy is play, a characteristic of the child" (Jung, 1921/1971, [CW6, para. 93]). In *The Aims of Psychotherapy*, pre-empting Winnicott, Jung added that the creative ability to imagine "frees man from his bondage to the 'nothing but' and raises him the status of one who plays. As Schiller said, man is completely human only when he is at play" (Jung, 1931/1966, p. 46 [CW16, para. 98]).

Moreover, Jung in *Answer to Job* did not conceptualise fantasies as a sign of psychopathology. He believed that "Visions, like dreams, are unusual but quite natural occurrences which can be designated as 'pathological' only when their morbid nature has been proved" (Jung, 1952/1969, p. 420 [CW11, para. 665]).[1]

For Jung fantasies can also act like a portal to the dead who are still speaking to us (Hillman and Shamdasani, 2013). During Jung's confrontation with the unconscious he had numerous encounters with different figures – amongst them were the persistent appearance of those he called the "dead." In Part III of *The Red Book – Scrutinies*, Jung hears the dead who had "returned from Jerusalem." He gives their concerns meaning when he takes up their incomplete projects as subjects of his own psychology (Stephens, 2020).

A ballad of image dependency – Jung's statements about active imagination

Jung references to his technique of engaging actively with waking fantasies later known as active imagination, centred around a number of points which he repeated and expanded upon in several writings. The key points deal with the "why," "when," "what," "where" and "how" of this technique. I grouped these theoretical points into eight different themes which Jung repeatedly developed throughout his writings, both before he called the technique active imagination, and when he referred to his method by this name. I will present and discuss a selection of Jung's writings in chronological order on these areas. The eight points are the following:

1 Definitions and aims.
2 Similarities and differences to other methods.
3 Stilling and emptying the mind.
4 Giving form to the images.
5 The push and pull to stay with images.
6 From philosophical and artistic temptations to ethical obligations.
7 Positive effects of active imagination.
8 Negative effects of active imagination.

Definitions and aims

Throughout his works, Jung gave various definitions of active imagination, which described a spontaneous or induced meditative process of dreaming with eyes open aimed to foster a dialogue between the conscious and the unconscious mind for the integration of the personality.

In the prefatory note to the essay *The Transcendent Function*, he argued that the method of active imagination:

> [...] is the most auxiliary for the production of those contents of the unconscious which lie, as it were, immediately below the threshold of consciousness and, when intensified, are the most likely to irrupt spontaneously into the conscious mind.
>
> (Jung, 1916/1960, p. 68 [CW8])

The union of conscious and unconscious contents will give rise to a psychological function "the transcendent function." In *Yoga and the West*, Jung stated that the method of active imagination: "[...] consists in a special training for switching off consciousness, at least to a relative extent, thus giving the unconscious contents a chance to develop" (Jung, 1936/1969, pp. 536–537 [CW11, para. 875]). The phrase "consists of a special training" is interesting since Jung is saying that some form of direction is required (like in RED) even though he does not say what this training includes.

In lecture I of the E.T.H. lectures, given on November 3, 1939, Jung explained how "Active imagination is to be understood as a way or method, to heal, raise and transform the personality" (Jung, 1939, p. 174). While in *The Psychological Aspects of the Kore*, Jung stated that active imagination: "[...] is a method of introspection (devised by myself) for observing the stream of interior images" (Jung, 1941/1968, p. 190 [CW9i, para. 319]).

The above definitions are self-explanatory and emphasise how unconscious images surface when consciousness is relaxed and are aimed to integrate one's personality.

Similarities and differences to other approaches

Besides voluntary and involuntary waking fantasies, Jung differentiated between dream work and fantasy work, in that in fantasy work, the ego participates in the fantasy process, while in dream work, it does not. Jung (1916/1960) has found that using dreams as the only road to the unconscious was unsatisfactory in several ways. In *The Tavistock Lectures*, he also expressed a bias towards active fantasy rather than towards dreams since: "[active fantasies] contain much more than dreams do; for instance, the feeling-values are in it, and one can judge it by feeling" (Jung, 1935/1976, p. 173 [CW18, para. 400]).

Despite Jung's conflict with Freud, Jung nonetheless did not fail to acknowledge Freud's influence on his technique of active imagination. Jung emphasised in *The Aims of Psychotherapy* that the roots of active imagination were to be found in Freud's method of free association: "At all events I learned it from Freud's method of free association, and I regarded it as a direct extension of that" (Jung, 1931/1966, p. 47 [CW16, para. 100]).

Furthermore, Jung's new method, which can be seen as a sort of meditation, differed from traditional forms such as Advaita Vedanta and Zen, or other meditation practices. What separates Jung's method from all of these is the use of one's unique and personal experience of the psyche as the starting point, rather than proscribed or transmitted formulas.

Through his seminars of Kundalini Yoga in 1932, Jung commenced a comparative study of esoteric practices, focusing on the "Spiritual Exercises" of Saint Ignatius of Loyola, Patanjali's Yoga sutras, Buddhist meditational practices and medieval alchemy which he presented in an extensive series of lectures at the Swiss Federal Institute of Technology (E.T.H.).

In the *Psychological Commentary on "The Tibetan Book of Great Liberation,"* Jung described how Saint Ignatius of Loyola "also made use of active imagination in his Exercitia" whilst adding that "something similar was used in the meditations of alchemical philosophy" (Jung, 1939/1969, p. 496 [CW11, para. 793]). He re-iterated this in *Mysterium Coniunctionis:* "What I call coming to terms with the unconscious the alchemists called 'meditation'" (Jung, 1955/1970, p. 497 [CW14, para. 707]).

Nonetheless, both of them have different aims to active imagination. Jung argued that these meditative practices "are of value only in increasing concentration and consolidating consciousness," but failed to make "a synthesis of the personality" (ibid., para. 708). Moreover, while prayer undervalues the individual ego, meditation devalues the contents of the unconscious.

Jung underlined the fact that active imagination is autonomous and does not follow rigid formulas, as in other meditative practices. However, two examples in *The Tavistock Lectures* challenged Jung's tenets about not following external meditative points.

The two examples in *The Tavistock Lectures* concern a patient of his and the other was his own personal childhood experience. The first example concerned a young artist, who used to find it difficult to do active imagination. This man had figured out a way of how to do it by looking at a poster of a countryside view at the train station and imagining himself in the poster. In the second example, Jung recounted how he used to look for a long time at a picture of his grandfather at his aunt's house and he would imagine himself descending the stairs in the picture (Jung, 1935/1976, p. 170 [CW18, para. 393–395]). Upon reflection, these two stories put the starting point of active imagination on an external point or structure to which they were unconsciously attracted. These two examples also demonstrate that, in order to get in touch with the inner world, one can also start to meditate on an external point that one is drawn to, as is the case in guided imagery towards which Jung was resistant. Jung preferred to underline the fact that active imagination usually moves from the internal to the external.

Stilling and emptying the mind

According to Jung, some people have the ability to generate spontaneous fantasies while others require more time and skill to do so. Jung emphasised the importance of creating a quiet atmosphere in order to be more able to receive images from the unconscious. In a Letter to Count Hermann Keyserling (4/23/31), Jung advised the Count to "switch off [his] noisy consciousness and listen quietly inwards" (Jung, 1973, pp. 82–83).

Stillness helps to produce an "abaissement du niveau mental," a lowering of ego-consciousness, which is a required condition to catch one's interior fantasises. In his essay *The Transcendent Function*, Jung wrote:

> The capacity to produce free fantasies can, however, be developed with practice. The training consists first of all in systematic exercises for eliminating critical attention, thus producing a vacuum in consciousness
> (Jung, 1916/1960, p. 77 [CW8, para. 155])

The phrase "systematic exercises" in the quote above is reminiscent of oriental practices as well as procedures in guided imagery. Yet Jung did not clarify what these exercises were, where he had learnt them and why he did not mention them.

Later on, Jung specified his oriental influences when he used a Chinese term to describe this idea of letting things happen: *wuwei*. Jung was influenced by Meister Eckhart's approach which he describes in *Commentary on the "Secret of the Golden Flower"* as "The art of letting things happen, action through non-action, letting go of oneself" (Jung, 1929/1967, p. 16 [CW13, para. 20]).

Giving form to fantasies

Jung explained that one is better able to access unconscious images using different methods. The best references for these varied methods to access waking dreams are found in the essay *The Transcendent Function*:

> Visual types should concentrate on the expectation that an inner image will be produced. [...] Audio-verbal types usually hear inner words [...] which however should be carefully noted down too.
> (Jung, 1916/1960, p. 83 [CW8, para. 170])

Jung included the tactile modality as well:

> There are others ... whose hands have the knack of giving expression to the contents of the unconscious [...] Those who are able to express the unconscious by means of bodily movements are rather rare [...]. Still rarer, but equally valuable, is automatic writing, direct or with the planchette.
> (Ibid., p. 83 [para. 171])

In *The Tavistock Lectures*, besides repeating the modalities of drawing and using writing, Jung also added that "women sometimes do weaving" and referred to women who "danced their unconscious figures" (Jung, 1935/1976, p. 173 [CW18, para. 400]).

In *Mysterium Coniunctionis*, he described a rare method to accessing the unconscious, namely the use of "a musical configuration [which] might also be possible provided that it were really composed and written down" (Jung, 1955/1970, p. 530 [CW14, para. 754]). Although Jung wrote several times about Wagner's music,[2] he did not amplify enough how through music one can engage in active imagination.

In *Memories, Dreams, Reflections*, Jung also spoke of how between 1918 and 1919, he started making circular drawings, mandalas, which corresponded to his inner situation. With the help of these drawings, he could observe his "psychic transformations from day to day," he described the mandala as "Formation, Transformation, Eternal Mind's eternal recreation" (Jung, 1963/1995, p. 221).

Jung emphasised the importance of externalising the images arising from the unconscious in order to not lose their impact and to be able to go back to them. He explained: "There is a tremendous difference between intending to tell something and actually telling it" (ibid.). Jung was not satisfied in merely writing down his fantasies. He wanted to find a more solid expression of externalising his unconscious fantasies and "to make a confession of faith in stone" (ibid., p. 250) which led to Jung's building of Bollingen Tower. Jung's Tower, which was a house for "personality number 2," was also an attempt to get in touch and integrate his sensation function.

The push and pull to stay with the images

Jung strived hard to stay in the presence of images as they presented themselves, on their own terms. In the *Visions seminars*, Jung used the word "betrachten" which is the equivalent of the verb, to "look at," but it "also gives the quality of being pregnant to the object" (Jung, 1998, p. 661). Jung described how if one concentrates upon an image, it tends to "shift" and "it becomes pregnant" (ibid., p. 661).

In *Mysterium Coniunctionis*, Jung underlined the importance of keeping the image as it is and not to contaminate it with one's own ideas: "Above all, don't let anything from outside, that does not belong, get into it, for the fantasy–image has everything it needs" (Jung, 1955/70, p. 526 [CW14, para. 749]).

Jung was aware of the difficulties and resistance in staying with the image. He also warned us that one has a resistance following the fantasy since the "conscious is forever saying, 'Keep away from all that'" (Jung, 1925/1989, p. 36). In *The Technique of differentiation between the Ego and the Figures of the Unconscious*, he urged his readers to overcome the resistance and "to face the figures of the vision actively and reactively, with full consciousness" (Jung, 1928/1966, p. 213 [CW7, para. 342]). Jung insisted that if this active involvement in the fantasies does not occur and observes the flow of images passively, one is bound to remain unchanged.

From philosophical and artistic temptations to ethical obligations

Jung (1916/1960) underlined the fact that it is important to stay away from the temptation of prematurely interpreting the images and the need to want to give a good aesthetic form to the image. In fact, he warned against being taken by either "the way of understanding" or "the way of creative formulation" (Jung, 1916/1960, p. 84 [CW8, para. 172]). In the *Commentary on "the Secret of the Golden Flower,"* Jung stated: "criticism is still likely to start in afterwards in the attempt to interpret the fantasy, to classify it, to aestheticize it, or to devalue it" (Jung, 1929/1967, p. 17 [CW13, para. 21]).

He also added in that "Insight into [images] must be converted into an ethical obligation" (Jung, 1963/1995, p. 218). For Jung, knowledge acquired from the unconscious, in order to have any significance, must become an integral part of one's life and have to be translated into action.

In *The Aims of Psychotherapy*, he suggested against giving patients' paintings and drawings artistic value since the aim should be "the living effect upon the patient himself" (Jung, 1931/1966, p. 48 [CW16, para. 104]).

Jung preferred meaning over beauty. When he was engaged in his confrontation with his unconscious and asked himself what he was doing, he heard a voice saying "It is art" (Jung, 1963/1995, p. 210). Jung was surprised, and could not believe it. He later replied to this voice: "No it is not art, it is nature" (ibid., p. 210). Although Jung believed in the artistic process, he stayed away from acknowledging the aesthetic element of the final artistic product. He did not risk moving too close to art and farther away from science in his project. Jung defended his position against art. Whereas the artist gives public form to emergent collective images, active imagination gives private form to images, which happen to be more personal than what artists produce (Dallett, 2008).

Positive effects of active imagination

Jung stated that when he translated the emotions into images he "was inwardly calmed and reassured" (Jung, 1963/1995, p. 201). He added that if he had not done so he "might have been torn to pieces by them" (ibid.).

According to Jung, in *The Psychological Aspects of the Kore*, the "advantage of this method is that it brings a mass of unconscious material to light" (Jung, 1941/1968, p. 190 [CW9i, para. 320]) while in the E.T.H. lectures he stated that a "second personality brings about an absolute change in character" (p. 106). He also stated that since the patient "is no longer dependent on his dreams or on his doctor's knowledge," he "gives shape to himself" (Jung, 1931/1966, p. 49 [CW16, para. 106]).

Moreover, in the later stages of analysis, the "images anticipate the dreams, and so the dream-material begins to peter out" (Jung, 1935/1976,

p. 172 [CW18, para. 393]). However, Jung believed that the greatest benefit of active imagination was during this decisive rapprochement with the unconscious "the unio mentalis, begins to become real. What you are now creating is the beginning of individuation, whose immediate goal is the experience and production of the symbol of totality" (Jung, 1955/1970, p. 529 [CW14, para. 753]).

Negative effects of active imagination

In the Prefatory note of the essay *The Transcendent Function*, Jung explained that the "method, [...] is not without its dangers and should if possible, not be employed except under expert supervision" (Jung, 1916/1960, p. 68 [CW8]). There are different levels of risk. One lesser risk is that of not carrying out active imagination properly and thus not gaining the result one is supposed to gain for example, "the patient gets caught in the sterile circle of his own complexes [...] or [...] remains stuck in all-enveloping phastasmagoria, so that once more nothing is gained" (ibid., p. 68).

Jung believed that the "subliminal contents, when afforded an outlet by active imagination [...] may even lead to a genuine 'psychotic interval'" (ibid, p. 68). The patient's ego needs to be strong in order to get in touch with unconscious processes so as not to precipitate a psychotic breakdown.

The crux of active imagination is the word "active." If one remains passive, one risks being overwhelmed by obsessive fantasies, or even worse, translating them into action and becoming psychotic.

The low profile of active imagination

As we have seen, the few references to active fantasy or active imagination are interspersed in Jung's *Collected Works*. Jung seemed to have done everything he could to leave his discoveries hidden from all but his closest colleagues. In fact, he did not publish *The Red Book* during his life time. Two of his write-ups on his findings on active imagination, namely *The Transcendent Function* and *The Seven Sermons to the Dead*, were only made available in 1958 and 1962 respectively, although he gave copies of them to some of his closest disciples and colleagues. There were a few patients who actually saw Jung working on *The Red Book* prior to the commencement of their analytic sessions.[3] Although their case studies demonstrate clearly the process of individuation, they do not capture the original spirit of the workings of active imagination which one can now see in *The Red Book*.

In *The Red Book*, Jung gave an explanation as to why he kept his work hidden for a long time:

> For at least thirteen years I kept quiet about the results of these methods in order to avoid any suggestion. I wanted to assure myself that

these things – mandalas especially – really are produced spontaneously and were not suggested to the patient by my own fantasy.

(Jung, 2009, p. 245)

Furthermore, Jung chose to keep a low profile on his work in order to maintain his persona as a scientist. Freud had warned Jung that psychoanalysis had to be a bulwark "against the black tide of occultism" (Jung, 1963/1995, p. 150).

Notes

1 Jung is not the first to put pathological hallucinations in the same spectrum as normal fantasies. He follows the same thinking as Galton (1881) before him who viewed visions and hallucinations as common occurrences in society and not necessarily pathological.
2 Jung was strongly impressed by Wagner's work. In the majority of his writings, he referred to some character or motive (most often to Teutonic gods) and their role in Wagner's operas. Particularly frequent was the mentioning of Wotan. For a review of Jung's writings mentioning the work of Wagner, see A. N. Kovacev's (2009) "Return to the origins: Wagner, Jung and symbolic forms," *Musicological Annual*, 89–115.
3 In 1933, Jung published his first extended case study of the individuation process, *A Study in the Process of Individuation*, which is on Kristine Mann (Miss X), who painted an extensive series of mandalas. Jung also used Christina Morgan's paintings for his visions seminars (1930–1934).

Chapter 2

Robert Desoille and the directed waking dream method

In comparison to Freud and Jung, Desoille (1890–1966) is a lesser known figure in psychology, whose contributions of the directed waking dream approach definitely deserve more attention. Desoille's ideas about his *rêve éveillé dirigé* (RED) method can be found in five of his books, which he published between 1938 and 1961 and three others which were published posthumously. His ideas can also be found in his many articles published in *Action et Pensée*, starting as early as 1923, in the journal *Société de Recherché Psychothérapiques de Langue Francaise* amongst others. Desoille's theoretical ideas about his method underwent three major developments throughout his life in France. Desoille has explained the RED method from three different evolving theoretical perspectives, namely Freudian and Janetian (1920s and 1930s), Jungian (early 1940s) and Pavlovian (1950s and 1960s).

RED: from occult practices to scientific experimentation

The French psychotherapist Robert Desoille in his book "*Exploration de l'Affectivite' Subconsciente par la Methode du Rêve Éveillé*/Exploration of the Affective Subconscious through the Waking Dream Method" recalled being very much impressed, as a seven-year-old boy, after seeing a hypnotic séance during a fair (Desoille, 1938). He was also fascinated with the phenomena of thought transmission, the witnessing of cataleptic states and a piercing of an arm with a safety needle without one drop of blood (ibid.). This instilled in him the desire to practise something similar and at 12 years of age, he carried out a mind-reading experiment with a female friend of his, at his uncle's house. However, it was in 1923 that his intuitive ideas took a more tangible form when he met a woman with the name of Lucie, who spoke of an experience of a waking dream she has had. Lucie described visionary experiences similar to those Desoille had read about in Theodore Flournoy's (1900) book *From India to Planet Mars*. Desoille's interest in the imagination, like Jung before him, was very much indebted to Flournoy's work. Desoille asked Lucie to put him into contact with the person who had given her that experience, a certain lieutenant-colonel Eugene Caslant. The latter wrote a short book in 1927 titled *"Le Dével-opment des Facultés Supra-normales*/The Development of Supra-Normal Faculties" that emphasised the supranormal faculties, which he aspired to achieve through his ascension and descension movements in imaginative space (Desoille, 1938).

Desoille became a student of Caslant and worked with him for two years at the *"centre psychique*/psychic centre" (Fabre & Passerini, 2010, p. 170). Besides learning about thought transmission, Desoille observed other phe-nomena happening in these imaginative exercises which did not follow Caslant's occult explanations. Eventually, Desoille realised that when one had his or her eyes closed and moved in an imaginative space the person experienced a change in his or her affective state. Hence, he started to study his findings more rigorously. Desoille defined the waking dream as "an intermediary stage between the waking state and the dreaming state, be-tween the physiological and the psychical" (Desoille, 1961, p. 10). He com-pared this state to that induced by Freud in his early "pressure technique" (ibid., p. 21). Thus, Desoille managed to translate an occult practice into an acceptable therapeutic method based on sound scientific investigations. Desoille named his method *rêve éveille dirigé* after Leon Daudet's (1926) book *"Le Rêve Éveillé*/The Waking Dream" which is a psychological study of the waking dream.

Desoille's therapeutic method

Desoille (1938) argued that the best way to help the patient have a waking dream was to make the patient lie down on a couch with eyes closed and with a dimly lit environment, thus facilitating regression. After a detailed anamnesis covering all kinds of habits of daily life, Desoille would help the patient to relax. In his later books, Desoille wrote that if the patient had difficulties relaxing, one had to send the patient to another therapist to help him or her achieve a more general relaxed state before starting therapy.[1]

Desoille gave an *"image de depart*/initial stimulus" to the patient lying on a couch and the patient would let his or her imagination work on the stimulus and create an inner oneiric drama (Desoille, 1945, p. 346). Thus, the patient paused from his real life and entered an atemporal mythical one, echoing Coleridge's most famous phrase of a "willing suspension of disbe-lief" (Coleridge, 1817/1907, p. 6). Sensation of the stimulus would change to perception, accessing archaic memory, fantasies, repressed desires, and firing a creative transformative imagination. Moreover, since the patient is asked to voice out loud his or her inner visualisation to the therapist, the method forms an internal performative expression as well as an external performative narrative, an ekphrasis. This gives the therapist the possibility to participate in the patient's waking dream. It also allows the therapist to intervene and help the patient if faced with difficult moments throughout his or her perilous imaginative journey. The oneirodrama takes about 45 minutes from the two-hour-long therapy session, which is carried out on a weekly or fortnightly basis.

A personal mythopoesis

Desoille (1945) described three different types and levels of images that are met during a directed waking dream – namely images from the patient's life, similar to those met in dreams, fabulous images associated with folklore, myths, and finally mystical images. According to Desoille, the oneiric drama is usually made up of fantastical figures and theriomorphic beings that alternate with individuals from one's current or past life. The patient can move in imaginative space between the world, an underworld and an upper world, where present, past and future conflate. Moreover, the patient can choose to be anyone and everywhere, with no limits to one's imagination since RED violates the laws of logic. Desoille encouraged patients to face the things which provoked anxiety in them such as dragons and octopi. At times, he also asked the patient to imagine the therapist beside him. Desoille also offered the patients protective objects of *"caractère magique/ magical character"* to face the fearful situation. He believed that one has to speak to the imaginary with one's own language (Desoille, 1955).

The patient can follow a waking dream like the movement phases in a slow-motion film. In the 1920s, the German psychiatrist, E. Kretschmer, likened the reliving of past events under hypnosis to the viewing of a film and he used the term *bildstreifendenken*, meaning "thinking in the form of a movie" (Kretschmer, 1922, p. 71). However, Desoille (1938, 1945) underlined the active nature the patient has to show in a waking dream and to experience the imaginative journey with all the senses, reminding us of the sensory involvement in the Ignatian *Exercitia*.[2]

Desoille directed the patient to ascend or descend in the imaginative space. Once the waking dream was over, Desoille would ask the patient to write down at home what he or she had imagined and to keep track of his or her dreams as well, a procedure found in Asclepian dream incubation temples[3] (Meier, 1942).

Before the end of the imaginative part of the session, Desoille (1938) asked the patient to focus on the body, to listen to his or her heart beat and to become aware of his or her breathing while imagining that every part of the body was healthy. The patient was also asked to take an image of health to use in daily life until the next session. The latter was heavily influenced by Coué's suggestion techniques[4] which Desoille was familiar with, as he himself stated when he described this part of auto-training. Then Desoille would ask the patient to open his or her eyes.

In the next session, the patient and the therapist would look again at the waking-dream content and compare it to the difficulties in the patient's life. According to a French Jungian analyst Dr. Elisabeth Schnetzler (personal communication),[5] her father, Dr. Jean Pierre Schnetzler (a disciple of Desoille who later became a Jungian analyst), wrote to his wife describing his sessions with Desoille between 1956 and 1958: *"Desoille m'a prie de rediger le compte rendu des séances et l'interpretation spontanee que j'en donne*/Desoille asked me to transcribe the interview of the sessions and to give a spontaneous interpretation to the material" (my translation).

During this part of the session, the patient and the therapist sat face to face. Desoille did not interpret the content of the waking dream as psychoanalysts would do, but asked the patient to share what he or she thought about the waking dream's drama. He also asked the patient about his or her dreams in order to monitor the therapeutic development of the sessions.

Types of Initial Stimuli

After several years of practising the RED method, Desoille came up with six themes which can be offered as an imaginative stimulus to the patients unknowingly materialising William James' "requisite stimulus"[6] (1902/1985, p. 308) of tapping beyond normal consciousness. The six stimuli are the theme of a sword for a man and a vase for a woman (its purpose being to understand one's own sexuality); the theme of a descent to the bottom of the sea (its purpose being to confront one's unacknowledged characteristics); the theme of a witch or a sorcerer (its purpose being to come to terms with the parent of the opposite sex and the parent of one's own sex); the theme of descending in a cave to find a dragon (its purpose being to come to terms with authority and society's constraints); the theme of sleeping beauty or prince charming (its purpose being of coming to terms with the Oedipal situation) (Desoille, 1966). Desoille did not necessarily follow these imaginative stimuli in order and at times he repeated them and used other spontaneous images arising during therapy sessions. One of Desoille's foreign disciples, Dr. Duarte (2007), differentiated between classic, circumstantial and elective stimuli and the therapist can choose whichever is most appropriate. These stimuli are similar to those employed by the German doctor Carl Happich (1932), who in the 1920s utilised a number of predetermined scenes such as a meadow, a mountain or a chapel as a starting point for visualisation. However, unlike Desoille, Happich's emphasis was mainly religious and his method aimed towards spiritual integration.

Desoille, in his first book in 1938, also mentioned that one could use not only verbal stimulus but also a sound stimulus. He also included the sense of smell as *"representations olfactives*/olfactory representations" (Desoille, 1938, p. 87) as initial stimulus, which he admitted to having never tried. Desoille wrote of avoiding *"les excitations tactile*/tactile stimuli" (ibid.), but argued that it is also possible for it to work if used with caution. The similarity between Jung's ideas of different means of expressing unconscious images and those of Desoille is very striking. Moreover, Desoille (1957) used a visual stimulus to work with one of his patients named Vania.

This consisted of presenting her with a copy of the painting *The Woman and Death* of Baldung Grun which is found in the Vienna museum, to start off her imaginative journey. Visual stimuli have also been used in the expressive arts such as art therapy. Visual prompts are used to help "unfreeze" the patient, i.e., reduce inhibitions and liberate spontaneous imagery from the unconscious (Virshup, 1978; Silver, 2001; Nucho, 2003). Both Prinzhorn (1922) and Cane (1951) referred to the Renaissance artist Leonado da Vinci. The latter's source of inspiration was ambiguous visual forms, such as the variegated colours and cracks in walls or crumpled-up paper. Desoille's method of using pictures to start an imaginative experience has not been referenced in the creative expressive arts literature.

Movement: the heart of red

Desoille intuited that movement in imaginary space of a waking dream resulted in an emotional experience and thus saw its therapeutic potential: *"L'image onirique est tojours le signe revalateur d'un etat affectif dont il est l'effet/*The oneiric image is always a revealing sign of an affective state of which it is the effect" (Desoille, 1938, p. 53 [my translation]).

For Desoille, images gave form to emotions, and emotions lent a living body to images. Before Desoille, a French psychiatrist Teodore Ribot in his *"Essai sur l'Imagination Créatrice/*Essay on the Creative Imagination" (1908) had already stated that each image is accompanied by an emotion and a physiological effect. Current neuroscientific research has confirmed that emotion-related cortical structures and the autonomic system are involved when engaged in mental imagery (Lang et al., 1993; Kosslyn, Ganis & Thompson, 2009). From a different perspective, the idea of imagery and movement was also being discussed in the art scenes of the early twentieth century where aesthetics became a question of experimental physiology and thus a physiological aesthetic, especially in France through the research and measuring instruments of the French mathematician and psychophysiologist Charles Henry (1959–1926).

Thus, physiological aesthetics assert that viewers respond to art through exact sensations, proposing that art can cause the viewer physical pain or pleasure (Brain, 2008). These ideas were taken up by Divisionists and Pointillists in art in the first decades of the twentieth century. Desoille, being an engineer and having a scientific background, was familiar with the results of experimental psychology at the turn of the century. One cannot fail to notice the similarity with Jung's interest in experimental psychology in the early 1900s which influenced his "word association" experiment. Desoille became interested in the experimental research of Charles Henry on how lines and choice of colours in a painting created a different feeling in the viewer. The latter seemed to have influenced the choice of stimuli used by Desoille in his waking dreams to achieve certain emotional states in the patient or subject.

Desoille (1945) equated movement with *la vie* (life) and *la liberté* (liberty). The primary axis of all movement is vertical and hence descending and ascending; these are the most important motions. Movement in space spells metamorphosis. Particularly for Desoille, the ascensional movement is crucial and its frequency and quality manifest the degree to which the patient has been freed from his or her neurotic problem that led him or her to therapy. Desoille did not discover the imagination but rather the "verb" of imagination, i.e., when one moves in an imaginative space, one simultaneously experiences emotional and physiological changes in oneself.

Desoille's own waking dreams made him realise that moving up in imaginary space can bring feelings of happiness and well-being while descending results in feelings of fear and anxiety. The feelings associated with this ascendence-descendance axis are a mimesis of the universal human feelings experienced during dusk and dawn. Borrowing ideas from the Swiss historian Jacob Burckhardt's (1818–1897) solar mythological imagery, Desoille (1938) explained how during dawn one tends to feel hopeful and positive, while dusk is usually associated with heaviness and dark moods. This is reflected linguistically in expressions such as "feeling down" and "feeling high." Desoille also found that movement from left to right can also have the same effect as if moving from a downward to an upward position. He seems to be suggesting an archetypal root to this physiological reaction. In his study of religious symbolism, Mircea Eliade, a Romanian philosopher and historian of religion (1957/1960), gave considerable evidence of the positive valuing of up and the negative associations of down in the beliefs and myths of Western as well as Eastern cultures. Eliade (1948, 1951) mentioned several impressive examples to support the claim of universality of valuing up rather than down. However, Desoille's discovery of a therapeutic effect linked to a motion along a vertical axis seemed to be more a result of a cultural-psychological expression.

Desoille's cosmology of heaven and hell

Desoille recommended beginning with the images of ascension which he associated with sublimation and evocation of the person's higher ethical and spiritual tendencies; this, he recommended, should be followed by a courageous descent into the depths like Homer, Virgil and Dante did before him. The images of ascent frequently lead one to encounters with archetypal celestial beings, irrespective of one's religious beliefs, and finally to experiences of a mystical nature, where the subject merges with, or is surrounded by light. On the highest level, the light becomes extremely white, and the images lose their outline as they dissolve into an all-encompassing light (Desoille, 1931). The ascent is experienced as a physical elevation and a moral one leading to a conversion to an ethereal state. He compared this upward-downward movement with Dante's opus of *The Divine Comedy* which can be seen as a long waking dream with a regression into Hell and a progression via Purgatory to Paradise: "*Cette association, que l'on trouve chez Dante, est l'axe meme de notre technique*/This association, that one finds in Dante, is the same axis of our technique" (Desoille, 1938, p. 90 [my translation]).

Desoille and philosophy

Furthermore, Desoille's method finds a philosophical resonance in the work of the French philosopher Gaston Bachelard (1884–1962). Bachelard is to Desoille what Henri Corbin is to Jung. Bachelard devoted his later writings to a series of studies on the origin of creative imagination. Bachelard's phenomenology refers to the creative imagination as *reverie* which connotes a re-creation of reality and not a representation. He dedicated the fourth chapter of his 1943 book titled *"L'Air et les songes – Essai sur l'Imagination du Mouvement*/Air and Dreams – Essay on the Imagination of Movement" to the works of Desoille. Bachelard argued that Desoille's method, contrary to the psychoanalytic method, offers "une mise en marche/a way forward" (Bachelard, 1943, pp. 130–145). Moreover, Bachelard named Desoille's psychology *"psychologie ascensionelle*/an ascensional psychology" (ibid., p. 21). In his work *The Flame of a Candle* (1961), Bachelard described imagination as the flame of the psyche, while in *The Poetics of Fire* (1988) he chose fire as the physical element associated with the imagination. Gaston Bachelard's disciples such as Gilbert Durand (1960/1999), Jean Jacques Wunenburger (1993) and Paul Ricoeur (1991) continue to establish a fundamental philosophy of the imagination which manages to transcend Sartre's earlier, rather dubious value of the imagination.

Desoille seems to have had a good mentor in the other French philosopher Gabriel Marcel.[7] Marcel is as important and as close to Desoille as William James had been to Jung. Lucie Desoille and Jacqueline Marcel were very good friends. Desoille acted as the witness of the marriage of Marcel's adopted son to Anne Marcel (personal communication).[8] Marcel mentioned Desoille in the third chapter "The Need for Transcendence" of his 1951 book *The Mystery of Being: 1948–1950*. Marcel also positively reviewed Desoille's 1938 book in the 1938 journal "*La Vie Intellectuelle/ The Intellectual Life,*" a Catholic journal which is aimed to reinvigorate Catholic thought in the wake of the successive controversies of modernism. Marcel, as a French existentialist philosopher and a converted catholic, formed part of the philosophical movement *le personnalisme* whose main preoccupation was to assert the inalienable dignity of the human person in an age which treated men as a commodity of government and the market. Marcel was also involved in the early 1930s together with Pere Amiable, the Swiss Spoerri and Robert Desoille, in the "French Oxford movement"[9] or "Moral Re-Armament" (Lubac, Rougier & Sales, 1985, pp. 42–43). The latter referred to a Christian organisation founded by the American Dr. Frank Buchman that believed that the root of all problems was the personal problems of selfishness and that the answer was to surrender their lives over to God's Plan. These Catholic values influenced Desoille greatly and were the basis of the philosophy of his waking dream method which aimed to free man to be of service to others. Furthermore, Desoille and his brother Henri were also involved in the worker's union. With the advent of the Great Depression which hits France in 1931, the political climate saw the unity of working-class parties fighting for their rights with massive strikes which culminated in the *Matignon Agreements*[10] in 1938 (Bronner, 1992). However, with the consequences of the Second World War, Desoille started to believe that only a Marxist ideology could lift the workers' dignity and moved away from a personalist-existential perspective.

First é is missing in veille

During Desoille's life time, in the early twentieth century, psychoanalysis was still not widely diffused in France since the French were not so keen on being influenced by the Austrian Freud (Germany was considered a national enemy) and were still trying to reconcile Freud's view of sexuality with their Catholic heritage.

Desoille invented a method built on the previous main therapeutic methods known in France of the twentieth century, namely hypnosis and the ideas of psychoanalysis that were slowly entering France. Desoille knew several psychoanalysts including Rene Laforgue, Juliette Favez-Boutonnier, Georges Mauco, Francoise Dolto, Daniel Lagache, Paul Schiff and Louis Beirnaert, amongst others (mainly those who later sided with Daniel Lagache and Jacques Lacan against Sacha Nacht and Serge Lebovici when the split of the psychoanalytic Parisian society occurred in the 50s [de Mijolla, 2012]). He wanted to develop a method where the patient remembered what happens to him or her during the session unlike hypnosis and in which the patient co-operates rather than succumbs to the therapist's control.

Desoille realised that in psychoanalysis the emphasis is on the past rather than the future and on trying to cure neurosis, while in his method, like in Jung's, he was more interested in the development of one's personality. Desoille (1945) saw his method as a teaching of the art of living which is open to all ages. Moreover, he argued that the waking dream method is better than psychoanalysis since the patient is less resistant to be open. Patients experience a "dis-inhibition effect" when they try RED. The RED method, unlike psychoanalysis, is built more on by-passing the resistance rather than on insight. This makes Desoille one of the first therapists to use the notion of brief dynamic therapy even prior to French and Alexander's brief-dynamic approach (French & Alexander, 1946).

Yet, Desoille did use certain key concepts of psychoanalysis. He borrowed basic Freudian psychoanalytic concepts of the 1940s and made use of the psychoanalytic terminology of the unconscious, the id, the ego and the super-ego. Although Desoille did refer to the unconscious in his earlier works of 1938 and 1945, he preferred to use Andre Lamouche's term, "levels of consciousness," in his later works.

However, Desoille moved away from three main psychoanalytic principles, namely those of transference, neutrality, frequency, and length of sessions. Desoille devised a new method of overcoming the neurosis and did not focus on transference for its resolution. Nonetheless, he still used the concept of transference by stating that the transferential relationship that the patient brings from the past onto the therapist is transferred to the images of the waking dream. Desoille also described a different view of resistance which can be observed via the quality of images which the patient brings up.[11]

Desoille also broke the cardinal rule of neutrality and exchanged it with directivity, thus bringing a somewhat relational stance to the therapy. He did intervene in the waking dream of his patient but kept an equal relationship between therapist and patient, unlike in hypnosis. In his 1938 book, he made reference to the French psychiatrist, Pierre Janet, who found that a technique of substituting one image for another is effective in his efforts to overcome the *idées fixes* of hysterical patients (Janet, 1898).

Desoille (1938) claimed that the only suggestion is that of going upwards and downwards in imaginative space. He recommended prudence in giving suggestions and argued that the therapist has to have his or her own personal therapeutic journey so as not to influence the patient with their own blind spots. The element of directivity caused a lot of polarity during his time and was the result of a heated controversy. In fact, a theoretical debate ensued between Robert Desoille's *rêve éveillé dirigé* and Dr. Andres' Arthus[12] "*rêve éveillé libre*/free waking dream," in the journal *Action et Pensée* of March 1956 (Arthus, 1956; Desoille 1956).

However, the concept which Desoille expanded from psychoanalysis is that of sublimation, giving it a broader meaning. For Freud sublimation consists: "in the instinct directing itself towards an aim other than, and remote from that of sexual satisfaction" (Freud, 1914, p. 94). Desoille realised that the concept was not well developed, a point which Laplanche and Pontalis (1973, p. 433) were forced to repeat when stating that the concept of sublimation still carries a lack of coherent theory. While for psychoanalysis higher artistic, social and spiritual activities are usually sublimations of primitive sexual and aggressive drives (Segal, 1952), Desoille, like Jung, considered that these same impulses and desires can also exist in their own right and can develop irrespectively of the satisfaction of the erotic and aggressive drives. For Desoille, Freud failed to explain how such transformation of impulses can be done, something which the RED method described very well. Desoille's idea of sublimation is built on Edouard Le Roy's notion of "hominsation" or "socialisation of instincts." Desoille believed that imagining oneself ascending freely meant rising above the concerns that limit one's daily existence and thus moving to a region of playfulness and new possibilities.

Despite Desoille's criticism of psychoanalysis which reached a peak in his 1950 book "*Psychoanalyse et Rêve Éveillé Dirigé/Psychoanalysis and Directed Waking Dream*," he still nurtured a good relationship with leading French psychoanalysts, especially before the Lacanian schism dominated the French psychoanalytic world.[13] Dolto (de Mijolla, 2012) claimed that it is through the work of Desoille that she fell in love with Jung's work (Arzel Nadal, 2006), and Favez-Boutonnier (1945) confessed to trying Desoille's method and was very receptive towards it.

Desoille and Jung: a Franco-Swiss correspondence

In the 1940s, Desoille developed his method into a full therapeutic approach and positioned it in a Jungian theoretical framework. This approach can be found in his 1945 book *Le Rêve éveillé en psychothérapie–Essai sur la function de regulation de l'inconscient collectif.*[14] In the third chapter of this book, Desoille gave a detailed theoretical account of a Jungian-influenced RED method. Through the Swiss psychoanalyst Charles Baudouin, Desoille became familiar with the works of Carl Jung which were being translated (without any chronological order) into French. In his 1945 book, Desoille referenced six of Jung's writings, i.e., "*L'Inconscient dans la Vie Psychique Normale et Abnormal*/The Unconscious in Normal and Abnormal Psychic Life" (1928), "*Essais de Psychologie Analytique/* Essays on Analytical Psychology" (1931), "*Métapmorphoses et Symboles de la Libido*/Metamorphosis and symbols of the libido" (1926), "*Le Moi e l'Inconscient*/The Ego and the Unconscious" (1938), "*Phenomenes occultes*/On Occult Phenomena" (1938) and "*L' Homme a la Découverte de Son Âme*/Man in Search of a Soul" (1944). Nonetheless, Desoille emphasised that his method was discovered independently from Jung:

> La technique du rêve éveillé dirigé a été élaboré independamment des idees de C.G. Jung don't je n'ai connu les travaux que longtemps après le debut de mes recherché.
> The directed waking dream technique was elaborated independently of the ideas of C. G. Jung, I came to know his work much later and after I had already began my research.
>
> (Desoille, 1945, p. 3 [my translation])

Despite Desoille's references of Jung's books in the footnotes, Desoille did not make any reference to Jung's technique of active imagination in his 1945, Jungian influenced book. It is only in his posthumous work of 1973, *Entretiens sur le Rêve Eveillé Dirigé en Psychotherapie*, that he made direct reference to Jung's technique. This is probably related to the fact that in the 1940s Jung had not yet published any direct writings on active imagination and in those instances where Jung referred to it, the works were not yet translated into French. However, Desoille made a direct reference to Jung's "Word Association Experiment" and he compared it to the initial verbal stimuli that he gave to his patients so that patients could engage in an oneiric waking drama:

> La method active, au contraire, ete introduite pare C.G Jung, dans un procede a l'abri de toute critique; celui des mots inducteurs. Le lecteur remarquera tout de suite l'analogie qu'il y a entre ce procede et celui du rêve éveillé.
>
> The active method to the contrary, has been introduced by C. G. Jung, in a procedure of inducing words. The reader can easily point out the analogy that exists between this procedure and that of the directed waking dream.
>
> (Desoille, 1945, p. 339 [my translation])

Desoille bridged Jung's scientific diagnostic word-association experiment with his scientific waking dream technique based on initial word stimuli.

Jung's archetypes and Desoille's chain of archetypal images

On March 21, 1945, Desoille wrote to his Swiss friend, Adolphe Ferriere, that he was in the process of setting up a *"société de la psychologie de l'inconscient*/a psychological society of the unconscious" (AdF/C/1/18).[15] Desoille's ideas incorporated both Jung's wider view of the unconscious and Freud's ideas of the personal unconscious. He believed that the imagery encountered in the waking dream dealt with a person's repressed instincts and unconscious conflicts, as well as with his or her undeveloped resources and potential. Jung's notion of the collective unconscious fitted in perfectly with Desoille's imagery encountered in the advanced stages of his directed waking dream. Desoille (1945) made use of Jung's theory of archetypes and the collective unconscious. However, he deemed archetypes as described by Jung, to be too static for the movement and transformation found in the directed waking dream (Lebois, 1955). Emma Jung, in her essay *The Anima as an Elemental Being*, wrote: "One does better not to picture the unconscious, [...] with firmly defined quasi-concrete contents" (Jung, 1957/1985, p. 49), thus contradicting Desoille's point. Desoille came up with the idea of *"deux chaines archetypiques de representations*/two archetypal chains of representation," one masculine and one feminine. Desoille explained how during several waking dreams the archetypal images tended to change. For example, in the case of males this could change from Satan, sorcerer, white magicians, angel and God, while in the case of female this could change from Lilith, all the way up to the Virgin Mary.[16] Desoille further explained that the reintegration of the conflicting images into their archetypal series helped to achieve a synthesis of the psyche and in this way it could achieve its *"function regulatrice*/ regulatory function" (Desoille, 1945, p. 325).

Moreover, Desoille made a distinction between "*symboles*/symbols" and "*effect-signe*/effect-signs" (ibid., p. 53). This distinction recalled Jung's distinction between sign and symbol. However, in the case of Desoille, he reversed the meaning. He followed the meaning of the terms given by the philosopher Roland Dalbiez (1936) that a symbol referred to a reflective meaning associated with a particular image which was given when the person's level of waking consciousness was high, while in the case of *effect-signe* the patient had to slowly discover the meaning of the images as they unfolded in the oneiric drama, which could also change according to the development of the waking dream (ibid.).

Desoille's model of the psyche

Desoille developed a model of the psyche represented by two concentric spheres divided horizontally by a straight line. The inner sphere stands for consciousness and in the centre of this sphere he puts the Ego (*Moi*) together with the Super-ego (*Surmoi*). Outside of the small sphere, he placed the personal preconscious and the unconscious which continues beyond to the collective unconscious. At the bottom position of the bigger sphere in his diagram, he placed the Id (*Ça*), and at the top part of the upper sphere there is the Self (*Soi*). According to Desoille, the Self, which for Jung spelled the totality of the psyche, meant to him "*un état limite de sublimation*/a limitless state of sublimation" (Desoille, 1945, p. 286). For Desoille, the Self was an expression of the highest ideal that a person can achieve at any given moment. Again, contrary to Desoille, Jung did not place the Self on top, because the Self can be approached through the body, i.e., instincts, or through the non-body, i.e., through spiritual impulses or archetypes. In his topographical model, Desoille presented a detailed explanation of the "how," "why" and "what" it means for the sublime to become suppressed.

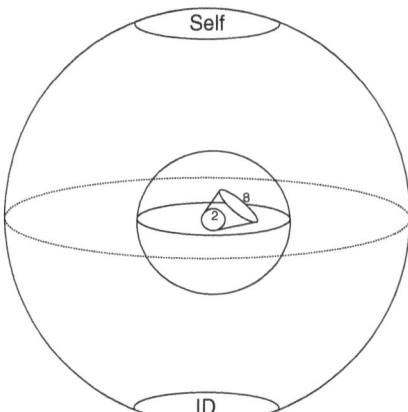

Figure 2.1 Desoille's model of the psyche.

Desoille underlined the unity of the psyche. The Self and the Id are considered to be the two extreme limits, opposite one another, and can never coincide. For Desoille, these two poles had an attractive effect on the Ego in the middle, which moves to one pole or to the other. The Self tries to get the ego to satisfy its needs (for the sublime and desire for development) and the Id, in opposition to the Self's desires, takes on the role of the repressive agent, exerting a new form of censorship, the repression of the sublime, i.e., the urge towards spiritual growth. Desoille argued that the repressive Superego should be weakened, enabling the subject to integrate his sexual instincts. The structure of the Superego has to be dissolved for its role to be taken by the Self. At the same time, Desoille goes beyond the Freudian framework in order to achieve the ultimate integration of the personality through a shift from the Ego to the Self as a centre of identity. Desoille believed that all feelings are susceptible towards an evolution which he described in Bergsonian terms as an *"évolution créatrice*/creative evolution." Desoille described the mechanism of regulation and evolution as the function of sublimation, giving it a wider meaning than the reductive one of Freud. Sublimation carries:

> *une valeur creatrice, et la notion de fonction transcendante, envisage par C.G. Jung et que le rêve éveillé met si bien en lumiere*
>   a creative value and the notion of transcendent function, envisaged by C. G. Jung which the directed waking dream brings to light.
>   (Desoille, 1945, p. 373 [my translation])

Desoille and Pavlov

In the 1960s, Desoille tried to update his therapeutic method with the dominant-rising Pavlovian theory in psychology, classifying his approach as a "rational psychotherapy." These ideas were discussed in his two books *"Introduction a une Psychotherapie Rationelle*/Introduction to a Rational Psychotherapy"* (Desoille, 1955) and *"Theorie et Pratique du Rêve Éveillé Dirigé*/Theory and Practice of Directed Waking Dream" (Desoille, 1961). Desoille dissociated himself from Freudian theory and keeps a few Jungian concepts such as the archetypal chain of images in his 1961 book. Desoille came to believe that the directed waking dream releases the normal inhibitory effect of the cortex over sub-cortical brain functions, and such weakening of cortical inhibition allows feelings to develop to an extent not otherwise possible. His use of "conditioning" and "de-conditioning" seems to be key terms in explaining the change of feelings and recovery, once images are transformed into more positive ones.[17]

Furthermore, the Second World War has had a strong effect on Desoille's thinking, especially the humiliation of the French defeat and the ensuing turmoil and instability in France. Desoille toned down the spiritual type of development and instead he focused more on the will. To some extent, Desoille was reacting to the war and the post-war period in France. Mircea Eliade in his *Journal 1* (1945–1955) wrote that after the death of his first wife Lucie:

> left alone Desoille finds support only in Communism. He preaches Marxism like a Saint Francis. He believes the Russian revolution will free humanity from evil, sin and ignorance [...]. He is trying to save himself by inventing an external 'mysticism.'
>
> (Eliade, p. 40)

Eliade's words were confirmed by Desoille himself in his correspondence to his Swiss friend Adolpe Ferriere in 1938.[18] His adamant belief not to charge for sessions also carried a Communist influence. Unfortunately, even though Desoille tried to modernise his approach by marrying a Pavlovian theoretical perspective, he failed to ensure that his method will become better known. In putting more emphasis on behaviouristic terminology rather than the fantastical oneiro-drama which is a hallmark of RED, he himself might have contributed to giving RED a lower profile than it deserved. In aligning his therapeutic method with a behaviouristic psychology, Desoille replaced his highly artistic and intuitive method with a more methodical one.

Notes

1 In his 1957 article *"Le Rêve Éveillé Dirigé Comme Méthode d'Exploration et de Cure Psychologique*/The Directed Waking Dream as a Method of Exploration and a Psychological Cure" and in his book *"Entretiens sur le Rêve Éveillé Dirigé en Psychothérapie*/Interviews on the Directed Waking Dream in Psychotherapy" (1973), Desoille mentioned J. Schultz's "autogenic training" influenced from Indian Yoga practices, which could help patients to achieve an optimal state of relaxation.

2 In the *Spiritual Exercises* of St. Ignatius of Loyola, the practitioner is instructed to walk into biblical historical scenes through the imagination and bring the scene to life by applying all his or her five senses, i.e., seeing the events, hearing what people are saying, smelling things and touching things – all within the realm of imagination. See *The Spiritual Exercises of Saint Ignatius of Loyola* Trans. by T. Corbishley, S. J. (1963).

3 Healing sanctuaries called Asclepions, dedicated to the god of medicine, were established throughout Greece. There, physicians (priests) practised a kind of spiritual healing centred around dream therapy on patients (pilgrims) who came seeking a healing intercession from the Divine Physician. The supplicant then entered the Abaton or dream incubation chamber for one or more nights, to receive a healing dream from Asclepius (Meier, 1942).

4 Autosuggestion is a psychological technique that was developed by pharmacist Emile Coué at the beginning of the twentieth century. It is a form of self-induced positive suggestion wherein the thoughts, feelings or behaviour of an individual are guided by oneself. Coué published his book on autosuggestion

in 1922 entitled *"La Maîtrise de soi-même par l'autosuggestion consciente: Autrefois de la suggestion et de ses applications*/Mastery of One's Self through Conscious Autosuggestion: Formerly 'Suggestion and its Applications.'"

5 Dr. Elisabeth Schnetzler attached to me a letter with her e-mail dated April 16, 2012. She quotes in her communication with me part of a letter written by her father to her mother about his experience of directed waking dream with Robert Desoille between 1956 and 1958 in Paris. He used to travel to Paris from Morlaix where he worked as psychiatrist. He also later tried this method with some of his patients and was supervised by Desoille. His daughter writes in this letter that her father continued to use Desoille's method even after he trained and became a Jungian analyst. He was analysed by Jungian analyst Dr. Arthur Arthus.

6 "Requisite stimulus" is taken from a famous quote by William James in his *Varieties of Religious Experience*:

> Our normal waking consciousness, rational consciousness as we call it, is but one special type of consciousness, whilst all about it, parted from it by the filmiest of screens, there lie potential forms of consciousness entirely different. We may go through life without suspecting their existence; but apply the requisite stimulus, and at a touch they are there in all their completeness.
>
> (James, 1902/1985, p. 308)

7 In a letter that I unearthed from the *Bibliothèque nationale de France– Fonds Gabriel Marcel* NAP 28349 (1–22) in Paris dated October 2, 1939, to Jacqueline Marcel, wife of Catholic philosopher Gabriel Marcel, Desoille (1939) writes that he was reading the work of psychiatrist Jules Seglas, student of Charcot, which Marcel had advised him to read.

8 In part of a letter sent to me by post on December 3, 2013 by the wife of the son of Gabriel Marcel, Anne Marcel, she describes that she had asked Lucie Desoille to be witness to their marriage.

9 There is also a connection between the Oxford Movement and Alchoholics Anonymous since several ideas of the Oxford Movement were absorbed as part of the 12-step programme of the Alcoholics Anoymous (Dick, 1998).

10 These agreements signed by Leon Blum head of the Popular Front Party, who won the 1936 election in France, changed the face of social welfare and ensured that workers had legal rights to form unions and bargain collectively about work conditions and wages. They also received wage hikes, a guarantee against reprisals for strikers amongst other rights (Bronner, 1992).

11 In *Exploration de L'Affectivite Subconsciente par la Méthode du Rêve Éveillé*, he observed three kinds of defensive images which are an indication of resistance and where he advised to stop treatment, namely *"l'images d'arrêt, les images deformantes, les images de refus*/immovable images, deforming images, refusing images" (Desoille, 1938, pp. 152–162 [my translation]). Desoille does not expand on the use and typology of defensive fantasies in RED which has a lot of useful clinical implications especially for diagnostic purposes.

12 Dr. Arthus had been a member of the "Charles Baudouin Institute of Psychotherapy and Psychoanalysis" in Geneva, who later trained as a Jungian analyst and together with Mme. Gilberte Aigrisse trained the first Belgian cohort of Jungian analysts who later founded the Belgian Society of Analytical Society keeping close contact with the Baudouin institute (Kirsch, 2000). It could very well be that Dr. Arthus had been more comfortable working with Jung's non-directive way of dealing with the imagination rather than with Desoille's guided approach.

13 In the 1960s, Robert Desoille was a vice president together with Juliette Favez-Bouttonier of the Societe de Recherche en Langue Francaise en Psychotherapie. The President was Paul Sivadon. The aim of this society was to gather various psychotherapy schools under one umbrella including the directed waking dream. In 1964, Desoille was in the administration of the Syndicat National des Orthophrenistes founded by Virel and Fretigny which later became known as the Syndicat National des Psychotherapeutes in which they tried to discuss the title of psychotherapist. The union was made up of various Freudians, Jungians, Adlerians and Desoille's disciples.

14 Desoille's 1945 book was reviewed positively in a philosophical journal *Revue Philosophique de Louvain* (Vol. 44 No. 2) in 1946 by Prof. Joseph Nuttin. Moreover, archival material from the Sorbonne University reveals how Desoille wrote to the Director General Monsieur Maurice Pradines of *Presses Universitaires de France* on October 4, 1944. Desoille describes how this book had to be divided into three titled sections and how he takes on the advice of the publishing house to remove the word *dirigé* from the title. He also writes how he has decided not to publish it in Switzerland hoping that his Swiss psychoanalyst friend Charles Badouin will advertise the book for him nonetheless. In another correspondence dated October 12, Mr. Pradines informs Desoille that his 512 page document was too large to publish and he suggested to divide it into two books so as to keep the price affordable. In a subsequent letter on November 8, the director informs Desoille that the book will cost 120 Francs and he will have ten percent profit from the first 1,000 books sold.

15 The letters from 1938 to 1946 are kept in the Archives of the *Insitut Jean-Jacques Rousseau* in Geneva with the name: Fonds A. Ferrière, dossier Ad-F/C/1/18. The letters sent from Ferriere to Desoille are originals but the letters from Desoille to Ferriere are copies.

16 Several Jungian analysts have written about archetypal images of the masculine and the feminine, such as Robert L Moore's and Douglas Gillette's (1991) book on the masculine archetypes *King, warrior, magician and lover* and Toni Wolf's (1956) paper entitled *Structural forms of the feminine psyche* which describes four archetypal forms, i.e., mother, hetaira, amazon and medium.

17 Similarities between Desoille's thinking and Wolpe's form of behaviour therapy can easily be found. Both approaches help patients to face painful feelings in graduated steps, so as to desensitise them from the situation which evokes these negative feelings. The two methods depend on the extensive use of imagery. Moreover, both argue that desensitisation is not enough and it is important for the patient to develop an alternative and healthy response to the stimulus which has, in the past, brought painful feelings or non-adaptive behaviour. Their use of fantasy, instead of being an escape from the world, provides another way of looking at it.

18 Desoille's correspondence to Ferriere on October 19, November 16, November 22 and December 2, 1938 (Archives of the *Insitut Jean-Jacques Rousseau* in Geneva with the name: Fonds A. Ferrière, dossier AdF/C/1/18) spoke about Desoille's critique of the capitalist system, the inability of the socialist parties to improve the situation and the need of Marx's philosophy to improve the situation. However, Desoille did not agree with a violent communist revolution, but more with an investment in education.

Chapter 3

Post-Jungian developments on active imagination

A few years after Jung's death the French analyst Elie Humbert wrote that in contrast to how it was during Jung's life, in the 1970s:

> The method is little used and is presented only occasionally in terms which render it either banal or esoteric.
>
> (Humbert, 1971, p. 101)

It seems that in Jungian analysis, especially in the developmental school, the shift to a process-oriented therapy lessened the importance of techniques such as active imagination.[1] In the last decade, however, there has been a resurgence of interest in active imagination with Murray Stein (2009) hailing active imagination as one of the "four pillars of analytical psychology." This interest has increased considerably with the publication of *The Red Book* (2009) and has helped to export analytical psychology outside Jungian circles.

Further developments in line with the classical approach of doing active imagination

Some of Jung's close disciples such as Barbara Hannah (1953; 1981) and Marie Von Franz (1980) wrote about active imagination. Barbara Hannah (1953) gave a detailed account of this technique. She also summarised when it is appropriate for the analyst to use active imagination. In fact, she recommended the use of active imagination when the unconscious is obviously overflowing with phantasies, when there are too many dreams (in order to reduce them), when there are too few or when the contents of dreams are inaccessible, when someone feels under indefinable influences, when the adaptation to life has been injured and when someone falls into the same hole again and again. Active imagination provides an alternative way for the analyst to help the patient to access the unconscious especially when he or she is finding it very hard to remember his or her dreams. It is also very helpful to overcome impasse in therapy.

Von Franz (1980) and later Dallett (1982, 2008), Johnson (1986) and Raff (2006) describe the stages of active imagination. These stages centre on stilling oneself to receive the image –externalising and dialoguing with the image, and living it in one's life. These models, while helpful for beginners, might give a false impression that active imagination is a fixed and simple technique.

Other Jungians add interesting concepts to active imagination, thus widening the meaning of the term. For June Singer, active imagination is more than anything else "an attitude towards the unconscious. It cannot be said to be a technique [...] because it is a different experience for each person who is able to use it" (Singer, 1972, p. 343). The German analyst Dieckmann (1979) saw active imagination as a positive regression since it sought a going backward in order to eventually go forward. While for Joseph Henderson (1984), active imagination was the central, self-reflective, psychological attitude drawing from the creative resources of human culture, namely the religious, the aesthetic, the philosophical and the social.

Several Jungian analysts have published books with case studies of active imagination made by their patients. Gerhard Adler explored a case of claustrophobia (1961) and in it he also gave a detailed account of active imagination through story writing and poetry written by the patient. Likewise, Rix Weaver (1973/1991) and Barbara Hannah (1981) gave single- and multiple-case studies of active imagination respectively. These works helped to demystify the mystery surrounding active imagination and made its workings more accessible to students in training and analysts alike.

The publication of Jung's (2009) *Liber Novus –The Red Book* has even made us rethink the procedure of the classical method of active imagination as we had understood it until very recently. In fact, Jung added commentaries after his inner dialogues (Stein, 2009) which did not feature in any of the steps given to us by Jung's students such as Von Franz's classification (1980), i.e., empty the mind; let a fantasy image arise; give it some form of expression; reaction by the ego, ethical confrontation and take it into life, live it. Yet, Jung's *Red Book* still emphasised that active imagination is a way of the solitary, as a personal meeting with one's inner self: "The touchstone is being alone with oneself. This is the way" (Jung, 2009, p. 330). Several post-Jungian writers (Chodorow, 1991; Schaverien, 1998, 2005) have moved away from this isolated approach of conducting active imagination and, in order to save it from oblivion, have introduced it in the therapeutic space.

Active imagination, expressive arts and expressive sensorial modalities

According to Whitmont and Pereira, the unconscious is "translated, as it were into a language of sensory images" (Whitmont & Pereira, 1989, p. 26).

Visual, auditory tactile and kinaesthetic therapies have flourished in the past decades and post-Jungians have been instrumental for these expressive therapies to emerge. Some Jungian practitioners developed active imagination into the therapeutic disciplines of the expressive arts such as: sand play therapy (Kalf, 1980), dance/ movement therapy – Authentic Movement (Whitehouse, 1979; Lewis, 1982; Woodman, 1982; Chodorow, 1995; Wyman Mc-Ginty, 1998; Pallaro, 1999), art therapy (Champernowne, 1969, 1971; Schaverien, 1982, 1998, 2005a, 2005b; Edwards, 2010) and body therapy, e.g., Bosnak's Embodied imagination (2007). These therapists presented active imagination in an external format and in the presence of a therapist. Yet the therapist's influence in these approaches is minimal and veers towards a non-directive stance. The role of the therapist is more of a witness to the unfolding psychotherapeutic process.

Jung himself mentioned visual techniques, writing and dialoguing, as well as movement. Although Jung did not make specific reference to drama as a form of engagement with images, he wrote about the use of dialoguing with personified images in *The Red Book*. However, Jung hardly mentioned music and did not explore the dimensions offered by the sense of smell and taste as entry points to active imagination.

Jung himself showed regret for not using music therapeutically since it provided a good means of giving form and expressing one's emotions. This is highlighted in his meeting with musician Margaret Tilly (1956). One wonders why Jung excluded the musical dimension in therapy even though in his trips he had witnessed shamanic chanting and Buddhist mantra singing. Music therapy and therapeutic voice work have been taken on board by post-Jungians. Some prominent exponents of Jungian music therapy are Alfred Wolfsohn, Lisa Solokov (1987), Paul Newham (1993), Patricia Skaar (2002) and Diane Austin (2006). Paul Ashton (2010) writes about the acoustical symbol first mentioned by Kittleson (1996), while Bloch (2007) develops Bion's concept of dreaming and extends it to music. Bloch defines music as a form of dreaming. Finally, Storr (1992) examines music from a philosophical and a psychoanalytic perspective.

Those senses which have not been written about much are the olfactary and the sense of taste. Maybe there is a case to develop the "third nose" and "third tongue," as well as the "third ear," (Reik, 1948) and the Hindu tradition of the "third eye." According to the French philosopher Rousseau, "smell is the sense of the imagination" (Rousseau, 1911/2013, p. 145). Psychotherapeutic work has repeatedly shown us how certain patients access unconscious memories accidentally in our analytic rooms besides being connected to the intuitive function. Moreover, smell also carries strong physical counter-transferential reactions as well as socio-economic prejudices in the consulting room, which have hardly been explored in Jungian literature. Patients from low socio-economic status can offer a challenging experience in the therapy room just by their pungent presence. Given Jung's interest in alchemy, it is rather strange that he did not speak about the moving power of smell and fragrances. Both alchemy and fragrance follow the dissolve and co-agulate procedure. Esoteric texts like Crowley's *Liber 777* (1909) have tried to explain the unconscious symbolism of different smells and fragrances. A Jungian aroma psychotherapy, as distinct from holistic aroma therapy, has not yet been developed.[2]

The same thing goes for the sense of taste. A verse from a Yoruba song titled "Hunger" says: "There is no god like one's stomach, we sacrifice to it every day" and Feurbach's (1862) statement "*Der Mensch ist was er isst/* Man is what he eats" gives us indications that through our eating habits we can also access our own complexes. Levi-Strauss (1964) in "*Le Cru et le Cuit/*Raw and the Cooked" explored man's cultural development from being an unconscious primitive man to becoming a conscious cultured one through his methods of cooking. Berger's (1976/2009) essay "The Eaters and the Eaten" has also analysed the difference between the peasants' and the bourgeoisie ways of eating. Post-Jungian analyst Susan Negley (2014) has explored the process of cooking as an individuation process. Marion Woodman (1980) has tackled anorexia nervosa from an analytical perspective, while Eve Jackson (1996) explored the symbolic aspects of food in *Food and Transformation: Imagery and Symbolism of Eating*.

Challenges to active imagination from different schools of Jungian analysis

The developmental school's contribution to active imagination has been more on its understanding of the possible dynamic roots and functions of active imagination. Michael Fordham (1956) pointed out the danger of using the term "active imagination" too loosely. He distinguished between imaginative activity and active imagination. The former strengthens the ego while the latter is aimed to strengthen the Self. Other Jungian analysts from the developmental school differentiated fantasy-related terms. Plaut (1966) argued that fantasies were not necessarily defensive or escapist as Freud believed, as long as the difference between fantasy and material actuality was preserved. More recently, Coleman distinguishes real imagination from fantasy which he refers to as imaginary. Coleman echoing Fordham (2006) states that the imaginary use of fantasy is a way of defending against a sense of absence and loss. Thus, its meaning lies in its defensive purpose, and not in the symbolic imagery that may colour its content.

Michael Fordham (1956) argued that it may be more important for therapists to become aware of when their patients are manifesting transitional phenomena rather than encouraging them to perform active imagination. The important thing was not the presence of creative imagination per se, but to allow and "hold" the patient in developing his or her own capacity to play. It could be a good starting place to develop one's own transitional spaces, just as a good enough parent provided an article for the child to use as a transitional object (Cwik, 1991).

As one moves towards the archetypal end of the spectrum in Jungian analysis, active imagination becomes the paradigm for the therapeutic interaction. This approach is called "image-focused therapy" (Hillman, 1981). In the Archetypal school, [3] active imagination is inherent in the therapeutic process. Archetypal psychology emphasises the need to "stick with the image" (Hillman & Pozzo, 1983, p. 54). Moreover, Archetypalists value the aesthetic attitude of images more, rather than the ethical one, and are less interested in translating images to waking life (Hillman, 1983). In *Healing Fictions*, Hillman argued that Jung's active imagination was not to be used as a "spiritual discipline, artistic creativity, transcendence of the worldly, mystical vision or union, personal betterment or magical effect" (Hillman, 1983, p. 60). He added that active imagination should be aimed at an ongoing self-understanding which "is its own end and has no end" (ibid.). Thus, Hillman put an emphasis on revelatory knowing and non-linear movements of active imagination. This contrasts with the linear stage models of active imagination addressed above (von Franz, 1980; Dallett, 1982, 2008; Johnson, 1986; Raff, 2006).

Other Jungians have also revised some of the notions that are inherent to active imagination. John Beebe (2010) emphasises the importance of the aesthetic attitude in the psychotherapy process since Jung tends to minimise the personal aesthetic experience of art involved in active imagination. Italian Jungian analysts Di Lorenzo (1970) and Donfrancesco (2009) write about cultural differences between northern people and southern Mediterranean people in how each relate to active imagination. The Italian analyst Silvia di Lorenzo explains how her Italian clients, who tend to be more extroverted than northern people, need more concreteness in order to engage in active imagination. As an example she would start from a dream they have had or use sketching of images so as to make interior images more real rather than expect the patients to dialogue with the great mother as Anna Marjula (1967) writes in her diary. On similar lines, Donfrancesco (2009) explains how Jung emphasises the meaning of the image (iconology) and its sublime quality as a result of his influence from the German Romantic Movement. This contrasts the Mediterranean iconophile love for the image itself which has a "presence" that reveals itself rather than being a symbolic representation of an ulterior reality.

Analysis as a form of active imagination

In recent years, other post-Jungians have used active imagination as a metaphor to describe aspects of analysis such as transference (Davidson, 1966; Gordon; 1968; Samuels, 1985), counter-transference (Cambray, 2001; Schaverien, 2007; Weiner, 2009) and even supervision as a form of active imagination (Cwik, 2006; Schaverien & Case, 2007). On similar lines, but from a relational psychoanalytic perspective, Thomas Ogden describes supervision as "dreaming the patient" (Ogden, 2005, p. 23). Moreover, even synchronistic events (Keutzer, 1984; Aziz, 1990) in the therapy session itself have been viewed as a form of active imagination since they can help in synthesising the patient's instinctual imaginal material located at the ultra-violet end of the psychic spectrum. This relational psychotherapeutic approach to active imagination arose out of a "desire to bridge the divide that has grown up between the classical-symbolic-synthetic approach and that of interactional dialectic" (Samuels, 1985, p. 204). Such views of the analytic situation focus on the analyst's attention not on solving the analysand's problems but rather on contacting and harnessing the power of a third presence. Both the analyst and analysand experience and receive information through the *mundus imaginalis*[4] (Corbin, 1972, 1983) while being immersed in the therapeutic space. From this perspective, healing comes not from the analyst to the analysand but rather from the analytic third to both. The analytic third is an autonomous entity that emerges from a psychic dialogue between the analyst and the analysand. The analytic field is evident only when the analyst and analysand relinquish the need to know or understand, even to know or understand whether the material is emerging from the analysand or analyst (Miller, 2004). Such clinical thinking brings analytical psychology more in line with current psychoanalytic relational conceptions of psychotherapy (Ogden, 1994; Mitchell & Aron, 1999; Loewenthal & Samuels, 2014) and even gives it a deeper meaning.

The application of active imagination to other disciplines

Finally, another group of post-Jungians have applied the idea of active imagination to several disciplines including cinema studies, theatre, research methodology, forensics, history and eco-psychology. Active imagination is applied to cinema studies in order to explain the effect of the cinema experience on the audience (Beebe, 1981; Izod, 2000; Hauke & Alister, 2001; Hockley, 2007). Enrique Pardo, a director of *Pantheatre*, influenced by James Hillman and Rafael Lopez-Pedraza applied active imagination to theatre performances. Romanyshn (2007) applies active imagination to the discipline of research methodology and he refers to this method as "alchemical hermeneutics." More recently, Daniels (2014) applied active imagination to forensic psychology and crime analysis. Active imagination has also been applied to history by Barbara Hannah (1981) who compared the dialogue between the conscious ego and the unconscious, which characterises active imagination, with the relationship Odysseus had with the Gods in Homer's *The Odyssey*. Ruth Meyer (2007) investigated how personal visions and dreams of several historians have spurred and influenced the direction of their historical investigations. Other Jungians have put forward a Jungian approach to eco-psychology that is driven by the principles of active imagination, which have been directed to the world rather than to the self. Psyche is not only inside the individual but in the whole world, captured in the concept of "anima mundi" (Hillman, 1982). This work has been explored by Hillman and Ventura (1993) in their classic work *We Have Had Hundred Years of Psychotherapy and the World Is Getting Worse* and other post-Jungians analysts such as Sabini (2002), Bernstein (2005), and Rust and Totton (2012).

The comparison of active imagination to other methods

So far active imagination has been critically compared to hypnosis (Hall, 1989) and to the imaginative component in E.M.D.R. (Tibaldi, 2004), while Wellisch (1950) wrote an article on how to use active imagination with Rorschach responses. There have also been a few articles comparing or integrating active imagination with the *rêve éveillé dirigé* method. In 1969, Rabassini wrote an article "*Osservazioni comparative su alcuni metodi di psicoterapia dell'immagine*/Comparative observations on some methods of imaginative psychotherapy," where he compared the directed day dream of Desoille, the Rigo imaginative technique of psychotherapy[5] and Jung's active imagination technique. Rabassini emphasised the need to compare these approaches, which were not widely known in his time, since he believed they are important methods for the exploration of the personality and can be useful instruments for psychotherapy. He compared the methods on four dimensions namely the role of the therapist, the problem of transference, the levels of consciousness during reverie and the clinical populations that can or cannot benefit from these methods.

The renowned late Italian Jungian analyst Bianca Garufi (1977) also wrote an article in the *Journal of Analytical Psychology*. For Garufi RED:

> [...] functions as a help and a guide in the treatment of cases which, to evolve positively, require Active Imagination, but where the patient is unable to use his own imagination constructively, having no experience of how to carry on a dialogue with his own unconscious. And it is precisely on account of this need for initial support and guidance on the road of Active Imagination that the Jungian psychologist can, I think, look on the RED as a valid aid.
>
> (Garufi, 1977, p. 124)

Garufi also stated that she used RED:

> [...] to delve, to fish at greater depth at a given moment, or resolutely to take the bull by the horns, or even make a break, a diversion, not, of

course, at a moment arbitrarily chosen but when the situation requires or lends itself to this variation.

(ibid., p. 226)

More recently, Annemarie Kroke (2004, 2013), a German Jungian analyst (practising in Italy), wrote two articles on how to work with active imagination in the analytic session. One in *"Studi Junghiani*/Jungian Studies" is titled *"L'uso dell'immaginazione attiva nella seduta analitica: alcuni aspetti terapeutici*/The use of active imagination in the analytic session: some therapeutic considerations" (Kroke, 2004), and the other one in *"Quaderni di cultura Junghiana*/Journal of Jungian Culture" carries the title of *"Brevi indicazioni teorico-pratiche sull'immaginazione attiva*/Brief theoretical-practical indications on active imagination" (Kroke, 2013). Kroke underlines the fact that active imagination in the analytic session can help the patient wean off the transference on the analyst and prepare him or her to be able to individuate. She also adds that the presence of the analyst can help patient when he or she gets stuck in their active imagination to see where he or she gets blocked and help facilitate the patient's continued relationship with the unconscious. She also describes how she is more aware to her counter-transference at the *"preimmaginazione*/preimagination" phase when the patient is going to enter his or her imagination. This allows her to open up the space in her unconscious so as to receive unconscious aspects of her patient. Kroke does not make any reference to Desoille or RED but she does reference the German psychiatrist Hanscarl Leuner who developed the imaginative method known as "Guided affective imagery."

There is a short dissertation by Zalewski (1971) entitled "Rapports Entre le Rêve Éveillé Dirigé de Robert Desoille et la Théorie de C.G. Jung/The Relationship Between Directed Waking Dream of Robert Desoille and the Theory of C.G. Jung,"[6] which could not be traced. There is also another short diploma thesis of the C.G. Jung Institute in Zurich by the Italian Jungian analyst Silvana Plateo-Zoja (1978) entitled "Analytical Psychology and Rêve éveillé dirigé." Plateo-Zoja attempts to compare the two approaches and argues that RED can enrich analytical practice especially when active imagination cannot yet be used. She gives a general overview of Desoille's theory by quoting from his later works and does not reference from his earlier books, especially his 1945 book which includes a strong reference to Jung. At the same time, she sees a strong affinity in Desoille ideas with analytical psychology especially with Jung's ideas of archetypes and the collective unconscious. She writes that RED is "[...] also, or even more a training the patient for more effective use of his own imaginative capacities" (Plateo-Zoja, 1978, p. 49). She adds "it seems that this technique is good in every case where the imaginative function is needed but cannot be summoned by the patient" (ibid., p. 55). Plateo-Zoja believes that RED:

May not imply such a deep personal experience as it is provided by Active Imagination, nor a real shift of the personality from the ego boundaries to an activation of the Self; but there are instances where this shift is not needed or even recommended. For example in the first half of life, or with borderlines.

(ibid., p. 57)

She concludes by stating:

My concern is the study of a method that is not Active Imagination but a technique of imaginative activity which, I feel, is very much, in line with the Jungian thought and can sometimes be used instead of Active Imagination [...] a sort of short-cut that suits the patient, enabling him to live perhaps less deep, but still valuable, psychic experiences.

(ibid., p. 58)

The Swiss Jungian analyst, Verena Kast, published a book in 1988 entitled *Imagination as Space of Freedom* on the use of guided imagery in therapy. She mentions the name of Desoille once but does not expand on his method or describe how it can be integrated with active imagination. The French transpersonal analysts Marc-Alain Descamps (2004) and Monique Pellerin attempted to include a transpersonal dimension to Desoille's method.

Notes

1 Thomas (2016) in her book *Using Mental Imagery in Counselling and Psychotherapy: A Guide to More Inclusive Theory and Practice* also confirms that there has been a wane in the general interest of mental imagery due to the postmodern understanding of the self as a product of relatedness and because of the relational turn in psychotherapy which has given importance to the therapeutic relationship. The one place where mental imagery is being developed is in the therapeutic approach least influenced by postmodern perspectives on the self, i.e., CBT and its contemporary variants. Moreover, Samuels in the chapter titled "Shadows of the therapy relationship" in the book *Relational Psychotherapy, Psychoanalysis and Counselling: Appraisals and Reappraisals* (Eds. D. Loewenthal & A. Samuels) questions what has become of one-person psychology in a relational era and suggests that "working with the private, a social imagery found in dreams and fantasies maybe a special kind of attachment" (Samuels, 2014, p. 188).

2 New cutting-edge equipment that records smell might also make it easier to work in a therapy setting through this particular sense. The possibility of smelling again particular smells can make it easier to reflect on the olfactory images one is smelling.

3 According to Andrew Samuels (1985), the archetypal school plays and explores images in therapy, paying the greatest respect to images just as they are without seeking an interpretive conclusion. The notion of soul, developed by the archetypal school, suggests the deepening that permits a mere event to become a significant experience. He first distinguished it from two other schools in analytical psychology, namely the Classical and the Developmental school. However, he revised this classification in 2015 and included it as part of the classical

or even eliminated as a clinical perspective. The new classification is made up of four schools which could be presented as a simple spectrum: fundamentalist-classical-developmental-psychoanalytic (see Samuels' chapter "New Developments in the Post-Jungian Field" in *Passions, Persons, Psychotherapy, Politics: Selected Works of Andrew Samuels* [pp. 201–221] published in 2015).

4 This term which means imaginal world is employed by Henry Corbin (1903–1978), the French philosopher and scholar of Islam. The *mundus imaginalis* refers to a realm produced by and in the imagination, it is an in-between state, an intermediate dimension, "neither one thing nor another" (Corbin, 1983, p. 1). Post-Jungians (Samuels, 1985; Schwartz-Salant, 1986) have taken this term and applied it to the therapeutic field between therapist and patient where images are drawn forward and can be accessed by both.

5 Leopoldo Rigo was an Italian psychologist who knew both Desoille's work and that of Virel and Fretigny. In fact, he developed his own style of working with waking dreams known as "*Tecnica Immaginativa di Analisi e Ristrutturazione del Profondo*/Imaginative technique of analysis and depth restructuring (ITP)" in the 1960s which brought the method closer to psychoanalytic principles of neutrality (removing initial word stimuli and moving upwards and downwards) and interpreting fantasy material from a psychoanalytic perspective.

6 The thesis could not be found in any research catalogue and when a request to Grenoble University was submitted through the reference department of the University of Malta, it was found that Grenoble University was split into various Universities, making it very hard to trace. E-mail sent to me on March 3, 2013 by Ms Kristine Saliba from the Reference Library – University of Malta.

Chapter 4

Post-Desoillian developments on the directed waking dream method

Desoille's work has been carried forward by some of his disciples, since in his lifetime he did not form any formal school. After Desoille died, his disciples formed G.I.R.E.D.D. – "*Groupe International du Rêve Eveillé Dirigé de Desoille*/International Group of Directed Waking Dream of Desoille" – in Paris in 1968. The first president of this group was Dr. Yvonne Fayol. During the 14 years of activity of this group, it started to issue the journal *Etudes Psychothérapiques* and also published two of Desoille's post-humous works. In 1982, the group's name was changed to G.I.R.E.D. removing the word *dirigé*, i.e., the directivity component, while emphasising spatial movement (Malan, 1975). This change was a result of a crisis where a number of individuals left the group. Besides, relational issues amongst the members there were also epistemological differences about the method. The differences revolved about the different interpretations of the processes involved in the waking dream method, the role of the unconscious, the importance of transference as well as the element of directivity and activation in the curing neurosis. In fact, G.I.R.E.D.D. was divided between those who were in favour of a straightforward entry into psychoanalysis, and "Desoillians" who believed more in the power of the waking dream itself. Some of the original disciples of Desoille such as Jacques Levine and Jean Nadal formed C.I.P.A.R.E. – the "*College International Psychoanalytique et Anthropologique du Rêve Éveillé*/International College of Psychoanalysis and Anthropology" which today is known as C.I.P.A., with very little mentioning of the waking dream method. Others, soon thereafter, identified with Transpersonal and Humanistic schools of thought (Dr. Jean Guilhot, Monique Pellerin, Dr. J.C. Benoit and Dr. M. Berta). Dr. Guilhot founded C.I.R.M.E.P. – "*Centre International de Methodologie en Psychotherapie*/International Centre of Methodology in Psychotherapy."[1] The first president of G.I.R.E.D. was Madame Nicole Fabre who remained president when G.I.R.E.P. – "*Groupe International Rêve Éveillé en Psychoanalyse*/International Group of Waking Dream in Psychoanalysis" – was formed a few years later.

The pro-psychoanalytic followers of the post-Desoille group formed G.I.R.E.P. in 1987 which still exists today and conceptualised the waking dream method as part of psychoanalysis. G.I.R.E.P. give their work a post-Freudian approach and remain the main, leading group in France. Revisions of Desoille's theory and practice can be noted. The initiatory stimulus is more patient-centred and is taken from, for instance, a particular dream image, a spontaneous image or emotion; an image from a test result or an image from a previous RED session. Furthermore, the focus on moving the patient upwards and downwards along a vertical axis is no longer used since the patient is free to choose any direction he or she is willing to explore. Moreover, the therapist writes *in vivo* the patient's waking dream. The interpretation of the content of the waking dream can be done collaboratively with the patient and special attention is given to transference and counter-transference reactions. However, even within G.I.R.E.P. several members interpret the method differently from French and British psychoanalytical approaches, such as from Lacanian, Winnicotian, as well as Kleinian and post-Kleinian perspectives. Another psychoanalytic school of waking dream is the A.I.R.E. – "*L'analyse Intégrative Rêve Éveillé*/ Integrative Waking Dream Approach" – of Jean Marc Henriot who was also a member of G.I.R.E.P. before he seceded the group. Unfortunately, besides the notion of archetypes, very few Jungian ideas have been integrated in RED by psychoanalytic groups.

In France, there are other groups, as previously mentioned, which have given more emphasis to the waking dream itself, refusing to associate with psychoanalysis. A case in point is the method developed by a disciple later turning dissident of Desoille, Andre Virel and his colleague, Roger Fretigny. They named their approach "*Onirotherapie d' Integration*/ Oneirotherapy of Integration," which they explained in "*L'imagerie Mentale: Introduction a l'Onirotherapie*/Mental Imagery: An Introduction to Oneirotherapy" (1968) and they had their school named "*L'Arbre Vert*/ Green Tree" in St. Jacques Street in Paris. They specifically focused on body relaxation methods, and believed that moving in imaginative space was more important than analysis of RED contents. At the same time, Virel was less directive than Desoille, and argued against suggesting protective objects directly to patients. Eventually, they formed an international association called S.I.T.I.M. – "*La Société Internationale Des Technique D'Imagerie Mentale*/The International Society of Mental Imagery Techniques" – which organised various international conferences.[2] Dr. Philippe Grosbois[3] published extensively on the method. Dr. Odile Dorkel-Drecq (Dorkel, Lambert & Virel, 2010) is responsible for the society. There are other active, non-psychoanalytic schools such as A.R.E.L. – "*Rêve éveillé Libre*/Free Wakeful Dreaming Method" – developed by the late Georges Romey and "The Imaginary in Action" by Dr. Michel Depeyrot. There is also the school of M. Oleg Poliakow[4] C.E.R.E.P.H.E. – "*Centre d'Etude du Rêve Eveillé en Psycho-Hypnothérapie Existentielle*/Centre of Waking Dream Study on Psycho-Existential Hypnotherapy" – that integrates the waking dream method with hypnosis and existentialism. Likewise, albeit in America, Schorr's "Psycho-imagination therapy" (1972) has also been influenced by Desoille and Leuner, but he has given it a Laingian and Sullivanian perspective.

RED's mild enchantment of the international therapeutic community

RED remains less visible as a method in the international therapeutic scene. Desoille's method of psychotherapy can be found in small pockets across continental Europe as well as in Southern America. During his life, Desoille lectured abroad and left some influence in Central Europe and South America. In his lifetime, he had a few representatives in different countries such as Dott.ssa Fusini Doddoli, Dott.ssa Secchi Belloti and Dott. Rigo in Italy; De Vriese in Belgium; Dr. Guillery and Dr. Bevand in Switzerland; Dr. Thomas and the Schultz group in Germany; Dr. Fernandez and Dr. Malpique in Portugal; Dr. Van den Berg in the Netherlands; Dr. Carcamo in Argentina and Dr. Berta in Uruguay (Sivadon, 1966).[5] Some of Desoille's disciples founded schools in their respective countries.

Desoillian roots could also be traced in the developmental history of the guided imagery schools in America. One Jewish student from Algeria, the late Colette Aboulker-Muscat, trained in Paris with Desoille for some time before the Second World War. She also introduced Desoille to the healing practices of a "school of light" of her North African ancestors (Aboulker, Muscat, 1995). In the 1950s, she emigrated to Jerusalem where she integrated Desoille's method with the Jewish Kabbalah teaching. Dr. Gerard Epstein (2000), the President of the "American Institute of Mental Imagery," studied in Israel in the 1970s with Colette Aboulker and then exported the waking dream therapy techniques to America which he also popularises with self-help books (1989, 1994) and teachings. Another of Desoille's disciples, Simone Blajan-Marcus, founded the "*Société d'Etudes du Psychodrame Pratique et Théorique*/Society for the Study of Theoretical and Practical Psychodrama," in Paris in the 1960s with Paul Lemoine and Henriette Michel-Lauriat. They gave it a Lacanian psychoanalytic perspective (Blajan-Marcus & Raynaud, 1997; Gaudé, 2006).

To this day, one can find other groups trying to re-enchant students with the RED method, in different continents. Until a few years ago, there was an Argentinian group called S.A.S.D.A.D. – "*Sociedad Argentina de Sueno Despierto Analitico de Desoille*/Argentinian Society of Analytic Waking Dream of Desoille" – directed by Dr. E. Rocca (Rocca & Villamarin, 2008) and another society in Uruguay which is still active S.U.E.D. – "*La Socieded de Ensueno Dirigido del Uruguay*/The Uruguayan Society of Directed Dream," of which Dr. Hector Anastasia and Dr. Milton Gagliardi (Berta & Anastasia, 2002) are active members. There is also the "*Istituto Biaggi*/ Biaggi Institute" in Belo Horizonte, Brazil, directed by Dr. M. Bernardetta Biaggi and individual practitioners in Belgium (Alain Feld) and Sweden

(Nicole Liljefors). In Italy, there are several schools of directed waking dream where it is referred to as *"Procedura Imaginativa/*Imaginative Procedure"* or *"Esperienza Imaginativa/*Imaginative Experience."* The Italian schools have kept a strong psychodynamic focus. They are namely *Clinica Rocca e Stendora*, directed by Renzo Rocca and Giorgio Stendoro (Rocca & Stendoro, 2001, 2002, 2005); the *"Scuola Italiana di Psicoterapia per le Techniche Immaginative di Analisi e Ristrutturazione del Profondo/*Italian Psychotherapy School for the Imaginative Analytic Techniques of Depth Restructuring"* founded by the late Leopoldo Rigo (1963, 1965, 1968); the school of the late Gian Mario Balzarini (1985) *"Analisi Imaginativa/* Imaginative Analysis"* with a strong Kleinian orientation which lost its focus after his death; and S.I.S.P.I – *"Scuola Internazionale di Specializzazione con la Procedura Immaginativa/* International School Specialising in Imaginative Procedure"* – founded by Dr. Alberto Passerini which is the only school accredited by G.I.R.E.P. of Paris and which is the most active school of the waking dream method in Italy today (Passerini & Toller, 2007; Passerini, 2009; Passerini & Fabre, 2010; Passerini & Vegetti, 2012). S.I.S.P.I. is also trying to give the waking dream method a neuro-scientific basis. In Portugal,[6] Maria Antonia Jardim, a student of Manuela Malpique,[7] teaches at CR.I.A.P. in Porto. In 2014, the *International Network for the Study of Waking Dream Therapy* (I.N.S.W.D.T.), which incorporates different schools of waking dream therapy, was founded by myself after organising the First International Conference on Waking Dream Therapy,[8] which was held in Malta in the same year.

Clinical applications of RED

In psychotherapy, guided imagery can be used as a relaxation for stress reduction, motivation for a more positive future, and to provide insight through exploration of possibilities and problem solving. The RED method covers all three objectives.

Desoille's books contain several case studies with different patients which offer a spectrum of different neurotic problems since Desoille did not treat psychotics. The case studies of Alexander (Desoille, 1945), the phobic Benjamin (Desoille, 1961) and the obsessive Marie-Clothilde (Desoille, 1971) are cases in point. Through these cases, he demonstrated that his technique is effective with hysterics, anxiety neurotics, phobics and homosexuals, as well as with cases of impotence and frigidity and with obsessives. However, he did not succeed in treating hypochondriacs and paranoids, nor psychasthenics.

Desoille's disciples and post-Desoillian practitioners have published several articles with different client groups. These include research on phobias (Bevand, 1961), anxiety (De Vriese, 1971), traumatic neurosis (Renaud, 1964), psychotic depression (Schnetzler, 1967), character neurosis (Rigo, 1963), psychopathy (Azevedo, 1953; Thirion–Henault, 1973), psychosomatics (Andjelkovic et al., 1983; Rocca & Stendoro, 2005), child analytic therapy (Mauco, 1953; Nadal, 1967, 1969; Fabre, 1971, 1973, 1974, 1998, 2002, 2004), sexual dysfunctions (Passerini, 2011) and psycho-oncology (Passerini & Torlasco, 2011). Current research has also reported positive results in its application to prevalent psychological difficulties such as P.T.S.D. and A.D.H.D. (Passerini, 2009; Valtorta & Passerini, 2015). There has also been comparative research between RED and the Rorshach psychological personality test (Dufour, 1962; Rigo, 1966; Maidi, 1983; Ternoy, 1997). Recent RED literature also focuses on the applicability of RED in couple and group therapy (Colette & Mesnil, 2009), brief dynamic therapy (Liljefors, 2009) and different cultures (Zanetti, Passerini & De Palma, 2010). RED is also being applied in education, to help enhance imaginative literacy (Lecchi, 2012).

Notes

1 Besides Dr. Jean Guilhot and his wife Aimee, active members included Dr. Deniau, Dr. Schnetzler, Dr. Auriol, Dr. Gerard, Prof. Mucchielli, Monique Pellerin Bougard, Edith de Vriese, Michel Le Guennec and Genevieve Lanfranchi. They remained loyal and defended the work as carried out by Desoille and were not in agreement of introducing the work as part of psychoanalysis.
2 The first conference was held in 1968 in Geneva; second in 1969 in Paris; third in 1970 in Cortina d'Ampezzo; fourth in 1972 in Portugal; fifth in 1976 in Paris; sixth in 1987 in Turin and the last one in 1988 in Paris.
3 Dr.. Grossbois was secretary of S.I.T.I.M. in the 1980s and helped to introduce this society in the International Federation of Psychotherapy in Rio together with the help of Dr. Jean Claude Benoit. He was trained by Virel and Jean Marchal. He worked with Virel till 1988.
4 M. Oleg Poliakow was a member of the original G.I.R.E.D.D.
5 After my research I added the names of Dott.ssa Secchi Belloti in Italy and corrected the name of Dr. Fernandes from Spain to Portugal and added Dr. Malpique to Portugal to those cited by Sivadon.
6 In Portugal, Prof. Azvedo Fernandez who knew Desoille and Virel wrote a book in 1975 entitled *"Psicoterrapia de Sono Acordado/*Psychotherapy of the Directed Waking Dream."
7 She was born in 1932. She worked in Porto as psychotherapist and teacher. She was a member of S.I.T.I.M. and studied with Virel in Paris in 1987 and served as vice president succeeding Dr. A. Fernandes (Cerqueira and Felgueiras, 2018). According to her pupil Maria Antonia Jardim (personal communication), they attended congresses in Brazil on the imaginary where she met Nise Da Silveira. She died in 1999.
8 The I.N.S.W.D.T.'s first international conference was held in Malta by the Malta Depth Psychological Association under the auspices of S.I.S.P.I., Italy and the *Ambassade de France* in Malta was called *Reveries from the past and Stimuli to the Future.* The second international conference was held in Milan in October 2017 and was entitled *Emerging Pathologies, Methodological Developments and Applications.* The third international conference "Between body and Psyche: the image" will be held in Paris in 2021. The website of the international network is www.wakingdreamtherapy.org.

Chapter 5

Jungians and the directed waking dream

Orthodox and unorthodox perspectives

The Genevan psychoanalyst Charles Baudouin (1963) writes in *L'Oeuvre de Jung* that as Freudians were critical of Jungians, early followers of Jung looked down on the element of directiveness in Desoille's method. With the exception of a few, such as Garufi (1977) and Plateo-Zoja (1978), it seems that the directed waking dream approach was not respected enough and was viewed with suspicion by classic Jungians and maybe not on par to the level of active imagination as advocated by Jung. The Belgian analyst Mme Gilberte Aigrisse (Feld, 1990) did not discourage a patient of hers to continue working with a directed waking dream therapist even since she could not practise it herself. In fact her patient, Monique Tiberghien, asked her for it after she enthusiastically experienced one session with another psychotherapist Andre Virel, a colleague of Desoille. Tiberghien writes:

> *Quand les images ont commence a deferler, j'ai dit ca c'est vraitement ce que j'appelle la psychoanalyse, c'est-a-dire le contact direct avec l'inconscient [...].*
> When the images started to unfold, I said to myself, this is truly psychoanalysis, that is a direct contact with the unconscious [...].
> (Feld, 1990, pp. 25–26 [my translation])

Mme Aigrisse confessed she did not know how to work with images on that level and directed her to continue to work with him.

Von Franz (1980) in her paper titled *Active imagination*, presented at Seventh International Congress of the International Association for Analytical Psychology, held in Rome in September 1977, criticised directed waking dream therapy approaches on three levels namely their:

a passivity
b use of the body and
c interference by the therapist on the patient's imaginative experience.

Her authoritative words seemed to have influenced the negative perception of Jungians towards directed waking dream approaches even though

Humbert (1980) questioned von Franz's arguments during the same congress. Von Franz's emphasis to practise active imagination as Jung advocated it tried to discourage Jungians[1] from seeking alternative methods in working with the imagination. Since von Franz was a highly influential classical Jungian, her words against directed imagery approaches have deterred Jungians to elaborate further the classical method of active imagination with directed waking dream therapies.

Marie L. Von Franz (1980) gives us specific reasons why Jungians should stay away from directed waking dream approaches. She speaks about the importance of letting the ego focus on the internal images without neither concentrating too much on them (since this may result in stopping the flow of images) nor concentrating too little on them since they may then change too rapidly. Such an attitude towards images may lead to passive imagination rather than a true form of imagination. Jung himself said in *Mysterium Coniunctionis*:

> What is enacted on the stage still remains a background process; it does not move the observer in any way, and the less it moves him the smaller will be the cathartic effect of this private theatre.
>
> (Jung, 1955/1970, p. 496 [CW14, para. 706])

Von Franz equated this form of passive imagination with Leuner's "Catathymic Imaginative Therapy" and Desoille's *rêve éveillé dirigé* (where she quoted his name wrong) and the work of W. L. Furrers:

> Nowadays this is widely practised in Germany as the 'Katathyme Bilderleben' of H. Leuner. Leuner took his idea admittedly from Jung and decided to simplify Jung's rather difficult technique, with a very bad result. I find it extremely difficult to teach analysands who have practised this form of imagination. The next step to a real imagination. W. L. Furrers Objectkivierung des Unbewuften, Bern 1969 (and NEUE Wege zum Unbewuftne, Bern 1970) stops short at the same point. So does the older technique of Le Rêve éveillé de René Desoille.
>
> (von Franz, 1980, p. 89)

Von Franz comes across as unknowledgeable of these European therapeutic imaginative techniques, since they emphasise not just passively looking at internal images like on a screen but a complete sensorial immersion in what one is experiencing with an imaginal-body ego. Such waking dream approaches can still leave a strong impact on the client and help him or her change aspects of his or her life.

Moreover, Von Franz failed to mention that in the practice of waking dream approaches, such as those of Desoille and other European practitioners, the therapist gives ample time and attention to ensure that the client is engaging actively in his or her oneirodramas. This would ensure that the client has allowed him- or herself to enter the imaginary space and is not making things up.

However, the French Jungian analyst Elie Humbert in his short paper entitled *Active imagination: questioned and discussed* goes as far as to question the Jungian dogma that emphasises the importance of focusing patiently on one image and not letting it develop into other images too quickly:

> What foundation is there for taking the image seriously to the extent of not letting it be transformed freely from one form to the other, but forcing it to keep itself in the form of concrete reality? [...] What does such a blocking of the image of the concrete mean? Does the role of both of them in the psychic not find itself modified by this?
>
> (Humbert, 1980, p. 137)

As we will see later on, there are different ideas amongst Jungians themselves on whether to freeze or free the internal imagery process while doing active imagination.

Another point raised by von Franz (1980) against directed waking dreams was the preparation of the body through relaxation methods before one engages in a waking dream. Most of the waking dream therapeutic approaches in Europe such as Desoille's RED, Leuner's "catathymic imaginative therapy or guided affective imagery" and Schultz's "autogenic training" give particular importance to relaxation of the body. To the contrary, Von Franz (1980) minimised the importance of preparing the body by relaxing so as to enhance the imaginative process. Furthermore, Von Franz interpreted the stillness and the lotus position of Eastern meditative practices as an externalisation of the inner stillness which one had to cultivate in order to receive images from the unconscious: "The outer 'sitting exercises' are only to be understood as a symbolic expression of this immobilizing of all ego activity" (von Franz, 1980, p. 88).

In active imagination, there is no specific procedure related to relaxation of the body that needs to be done prior to its commencement. In the European therapeutic imaginative methods, as in the Asclepian shrines of Epidaurus and Kos in Ancient Greece, the relaxed supine body is not absent, but a present protagonist of the relationship and provides a living stage for the theatre of the imagination to take place (Meier, 1949). Research carried out by Morgan and Bakan (1965) found that reclining subjects in a sensory-deprivation situation produced more vivid imagery than subjects sitting up. Segal and Glickman (1967) indicated that a supine position favours vivid imagery. Such findings affirm the importance of the psychoanalytic couch. Some French psychoanalysts, in the 60s and 70s, gave more importance to the relaxed body of the patient and invented psychoanalytic relaxation methods such as the "tonic dialogue" of Julian Ajuriaguerra (1959) and "induction variable" of Michel Sapir (1975) which seem to have been influenced by hypnosis and autogenic training. In *The Psychology of the Transference*, Jung writes: "[...] the body is necessary if the unconscious is not to have destructive effects on ego consciousness, for it is the body that gives bounds to the personality" (Jung, 1946/1966, p. 294 [CW16, para. 503]).

In light of these ideas, it seems surprising that analytical psychology has not as yet developed more systematic methods to carry out what body psychotherapists call grounding[2] an individual (Lowen, 1975). These methods are aimed at embodying the individual in his or her own somatic reality, which is equivalent to what Jung calls "living in the body." Jungian psychology shows a theoretical ambivalence towards the body, while ignoring its relevance in the clinical sphere. Jung himself believed in the unity of body and mind. His word association experiment at the Burghozli at the beginning of his career demonstrated that the unconscious complex has a somatic aspect located in the body. Overall, Jung's contribution to the mind-body problem was more philosophical and abstract rather than clinical. Jung still exposed his bias towards the ultra-violet, imagistic pole of the body-mind spectrum when he argued:

> [the] realisation and assimilation of instinct never takes place by absorption into the instinctual sphere but only through the integration of the image which signifies and at the same time evokes the instinct.
>
> (Jung, 1954/1960, p. 211 [CW8, para. 414])

Similarly, the blind spot of introverted intuitive Jungian analysts is their tendency to regard image and imagination as a more important dimension of the psyche than the body. Post-Jungians are attempting to address the somehow ignored body aspect in analytical psychology (McNeely, 1987; Chodorow, 1995; Wyman-Mc Ginty, 1998; Greene, 2001; Conger, 2005; Bosnak, 2007; Sassenfeld, 2008). The body can bring our psychophysiological experience to an emotional level of felt psychic experience, which can bridge inevitable gaps in being.

Desoille (1938) demonstrated through his therapeutic method the relationship between the mind and the body, i.e., during imagery physiological reactions such as changes in breathing and heart rate occur. Similar results are also visible in active imagination through movement. In fact, Wyman Mc-Ginty (1998) argues that therapeutic work with the body allows spontaneous access to the patient's early affective and somatic memory[3] without requiring conscious insight. Even sand play therapy (another form of active imagination) does not rely on the ego's understanding of the unconscious material projected in sand representations for individuation to take place.

Von Franz was also critical, besides the two already raised points of passive imagination and the relaxation of the body in directed waking dreams, by the direct interference of the therapist in the patient's waking dream. In this she was following Jung, since he criticised any attempt at interfering in the imaginative process of the patient: "Above all, don't let anything from outside, that does not belong, get into it, for the fantasy-image has everything it needs" (Jung, 1955/1970, p. 526 [CW14, para. 749]). Von Franz (1980) disagreed with those therapists who could intervene either by giving a stimulus (as in Happich's method or Schultz's advanced meditative stages of "autogenic training") or by suggesting a solution when faced with a problem. Von Franz reminded the readers that Jung would never interfere and would leave the patient to find his own solution. She mentioned an episode when Jung described the work with one of his female patients who in her active imagination did not know how to get to another side of the wall. She was stuck for a long time until eventually she thought of a hammer to make a hole in the wall. Von Franz argued that had Jung helped her, she would have remained without "defenses, infantile and passive" (Von Franz, 1980, p. 92). One has to face one's issues in the first person and with one's own efforts.

More recently, Dallett writes that when:

> The analyst's or guide's images are thus added to a patient's inner equation, which muddies the relationship between ego and unconscious and increases the ever-present temptation for a patient to put himself totally in the hands of the analyst, giving up responsibility for his own psyche.
> (Dallett, 2008, pp. 56–57)

Jung himself, in *Mysterium Coniunctionis*, had spoken against the prescribed formulae given by guides in meditation practices since "their purpose is to shield consciousness from the unconscious and to suppress it" (Jung, 1955/1970, p. 498 [CW14, para. 708]). Jung (2009) moved away from the idea of external guides and chose instead to rely more on his internal guide Philemon as he describes in *The Red Book*.

Despite Jung's overall consistency on the procedures of active imagination, his disciples did not seem to blindly imitate the procedures of their master and allowed for improvisations. Recent research by Wendy Swan (2007) has debunked the classical Jungian idea that active imagination should be practised away from the analyst. In her research on Tina Keller, a psychoanalyst who has been analysed by both Jung and Antonia Wolff, she claims that, thankfully, Wolff saved Keller from a menacing figure from the unconscious dubbed Leonard which she could not deal with on her own. Keller writes how:

> [...] one day Toni Wolff said out loud for the black doctor to hear 'if this man has a message for you, he must first translate it in such a way that it can be understood by a modern woman' as she said this, I had the impression as if a flash of lightening went through the room and I was free. The tension left, the obsession was gone and never came back [...].
> (Keller, 1981, p. 23)

Tina Keller had been engaging in active imagination using spontaneous writing which Jung had been teaching her. At one point, she saw Leonard, this male figure from her unconscious, who was acting like a conjurer and disturbing her. Ms. Keller was astonished that when she presented the material of active imagination she has had with this figure, Jung just laughed and did not know what to say to her. Antonia Wolff responded on Mrs. Keller's behalf to Leonard while Keller was undergoing analysis with her. In this way, Wolff helped Keller appease the figure of Leonard. This incident highlights the discrepancy between what Jung wrote and what he actually did. It also describes the importance of the analyst as a here-and-now provider of safety when the unconscious threatens to overwhelm the ego, and clearly demonstrates that a "healthy" interference by the analyst can at times save a patient's sanity.

On a similar case, Gerhard Adler (1957), in his book "*Etudes de Psychologie Jungienne*/Studies of Analytical Psychology," describes a case of a woman who was an insomniac. She was afraid of a grey figure who appeared in her imagination as soon as she was about to sleep. Adler described how at one point in therapy he took a risk by asking her to directly describe to him this figure, as well as give him its name. After some resistance, the patient described the figure as a female person named like her. She broke into tears as she experienced the confrontation spurned by the therapist. This procedure seemed to free her libido from her autonomous complex which was linked to this frightening figure and she could thus integrate and acknowledge a part of herself.

According to Adler, the example contains all the elements of active imagination. However, it was more the analyst than the patient who confronted the unconscious of the patient (Adler, 1957, p 64). Adler also mentioned another case of a patient who was overwhelmed by the violent unconscious images she drew and had to phone him in order to rid herself from an artificially induced psychotic state. For Adler, it seemed that the presence of the therapist was indispensable for active imagination and for the dialogue of the conscious part of the patient with his or her unconscious aspects. He did not emphasise the weaning of the transference relationship before active imagination could be pursued in the absence of the analyst.

Jungians might have felt compelled to interfere in the active imagination process as Desoille described in a lecture given in January 1965 at the University of Sorbonne on his waking dream method:

> Jungian analysts are familiar with these images but only as they have arisen spontaneously from folklore traditions. They have no methods for intentionally evoking them so that they can be studied in vivo and used therapeutically.
>
> (Desoille, 1966, p. 25)

It seems that besides theoretical reasons to practise active imagination alone, such as to avoid having a contamination of the transference or a slowing down of the unconscious flow, Jung had other practical reasons that suited his needs. The privacy of active imagination that analysands were directed to seems to have suited Jung in such a way that it made it possible for him to cope with the large number of analysands that he had and that were coming from all over the world. It also suited international analysands that could not stay for a long time to complete their analysis with Jung. Douglas (1993), in the biography of Christiana Morgan, explains the latter when she writes:

> Jung cast around for something that could [...] engage the analysand actively in his or her own cure without taking up more of Jung's already overbooked schedule. He decided to investigate the possibility of active imagination as a clinical and therapeutic tool that an analysand could employ privately.
>
> (Douglas, 1993, p. 155)

The incidents above demonstrate that active imagination could be practised in the analysis itself and that the analyst can also use an element of directivity to help the analysand cope with unconscious threatening figures. This kind of intervening by the analyst is not really unorthodox as many Jungians and students were led to believe, and has a close resemblance to the directive role of the therapist in the directed waking dream method of Desoille. This calls for a timely theoretical development of how elements of the directed waking dream can be better integrated with active imagination, when practised as an integral part of analysis. Such a development could possibly have been withheld since the introduction of Jung's analytical psychology in France seems to have been very difficult partly due to Jung's fault and partly due to the French culture of the twentieth century.

The relational aspect in active imagination

Classical Jungian understanding of active imagination underlies the importance of the symbolic as well of the need to engage in active imagination on our own and outside of the analytic session so as not to remain dependent on the analyst. As we have seen earlier, before Jung coined the term active imagination, he referred to it as the "technique of introversion" and as "introspection." Jung (2009) presented an introverted view of active imagination in *The Red Book*'s confrontation with the unconscious which came soon after he ended the fatherly and somewhat dependent relationship with Freud. This subjective experience seemed to have coloured the individualistic focus of active imagination and the emphasis on independence from the analyst. Like an abandoned mythic child, Jung faced the dragons of the unconscious on his own. In moments of difficulty, Antonia Wolff saved him from being overwhelmed by the unconscious. His family and his clinical practice also ensured that he remained grounded in his life, when faced with difficulties. For Jung, in active imagination the space shifted from external dependence on the analyst to a more internal dependence on sources within oneself since "It is a way of attaining liberation by one's own efforts and of finding the courage to be oneself" (Jung, 1916/1960, p. 9 [CW8, para. 749]).

Von Franz developed further the concept of active imagination by applying to it Jung's typology theory. She applied the four functions to active imagination but did not go on to explore how the two attitudes, i.e., introversion and extroversion, could work in active imagination. Von Franz suggested very practical ways of how individuals and patients could tap into their inferior functions through particular forms of active imagination related to the opposite of one's superior functions. For example, intuitives could make use of sensate practices such as working with clay; thinkers could engage in movement activities or else make colourful paintings while sensates could benefit by producing fictitious writings (Von Franz & Hillman, 1971, p. 63). Yet she failed to mention how introverts could extrovert through their engagement with active imagination in the presence of someone. This notion is succinctly concluded by Jungian analyst Joan Chodorow, when she states that individuation through active imagination requires "learning to be oneself in the presence of another. For others it is important to work alone. Everyone is unique" (Chodorow, 1997, p. 17). This issue is also raised by another of Jung's disciples, Elie Humbert, but it is not until later that post-Jungians give a relational approach to active imagination, making it more accessible amongst analysts.

Jungian analyst Elie Humbert questions the isolation in relation to the other person in active imagination, since images can lead to satisfaction of desires as well as to a risk of overwhelming the patient:

> We speak of Eros, and practice shows that in fact active imagination supports and develops it. But what Eros are we talking about where the other person is not present? Is not active imagination a dangerously glib exercise since the affects take shape there outside of all relation to the object?
>
> (Humbert, 1980, p. 136)

Moreover, Humbert (1979) in his paper "*Il ruolo dell'immagine nella psicologia analitica/* The role of the imagination in analytical psychology" adds that the patient during active imagination runs the risk of remaining in a narcissistic shell or under the spell of the mother. This danger is more pronounced in analytical psychology since the notion of subjectivity is derived through a confrontation with the unconscious, which ultimately remains an intrapsychic and endogenous thing, while for Freudians subjectivity emerges from a resolution of the oedipal complex. He also adds that the objectivity met through the collective unconscious in dreams and imagery is not the same as the external reality:

> *Non si puo' condurre l'analisi soltanto nella prospettiva degli archetipi, ma anche in quella delle pulsioni e del linguaggio.*
> One cannot conduct analysis solely by just focusing on archetypes but one also has to take into account impulses and language.
> (Humbert, 1979, p. 8 [my translation])

Post-Jungians have developed forms of active imagination that support regression through expressive arts methods, in which the therapist acts as a witness to the spontaneous emerging process in which the patient engages in, such as movement, sand play or drawing. The purpose of the therapist during different forms of active imagination is to serve as a witness, as well as to create a sense of trust, of emotional attunement, such that early states of mind can emerge and become known in the context of a relationship between two people. The therapist is more of a presence than a guide. During active imagination, the images from the unconscious, encountered by the ego, can begin to link up powerful feelings that are difficult to hold onto. The therapist can help to metabolise the intensity of the affects and manage the psychic pain which has been stored in the body. Research in attachment (Fonagy, 2001) suggests that symbolic representation is achieved when there is adequate mirroring, and a sense of containment on the part of the caregiver or analyst in our case. This is especially important when working with patients whose attachment relationships have been damaged.

Nonetheless, post-Jungians (with the exception of Garufi, 1977; Plateo Zoja, 1978; and Kroke, 2004, 2013) have hardly made reference to visualisation in therapy with the patient lying down and in the presence of a more active therapist. If active imagination is practised in the session during analysis, RED can offer other ideas to the practitioner of how to work in this context. The implications of active imagination vis-à-vis the "other's" role have thus to be reversed, as in RED. The power of the work done through active imagination can be deepened with the therapist as a guide facilitating the process, bearing witness and beholding a safe and sacred space for the supine patient. The therapist or guide, like a Brechtian theatre director, is a witness of the carrying out of the patient's ethical obligations of the waking dream in his or her life.

RED is carried out with one patient at a time in the presence of a therapist (a co-therapist might be present to lessen transference complications). Desoille, unlike Assogioli, does not come up with group fantasies which have become popular in the U.S.A. and amongst humanistic therapists.

However, a disciple of Desoille, Leopoldo Rigo, one of the pioneers of the *Rêve éveillé* in Italy (Rigo-Uberto, 1966–1967; Rigo, 1970), develops it along Kleinian lines and extends Desoille's imagery techniques to group treatment.[4]

Such relational versions of active imagination, despite keeping its personal development focus, move closer to the personal-social focus continuum of oneiric therapeutic techniques, such as van Loben Sels' (2003) method of "dreaming-in-the-world," or to the more known approach of "social dreaming" (Lawrence, 2003). The latter approaches seem to be motivated by the belief that the unconscious nowadays reigns in the "polis" (Hillman, 1994, p. 30) and that therapy has to help us look at collective issues that we try to look away from by indulging unconsciously in a materialistic world of consumption. Such approaches aim to sensitise us towards our indifference to the world and our current existential alienation.

Notes

1 In fact, Garufi's article and Plateo-Zoja's thesis (which also references the 1977 Rome congress and Garufi's own article on the RED method) are unique attempts to break away from an orthodox mentality in analytical psychology. Both Italian contributions were written in the wake of the debate that arose in the congress in Italy, and sound more conciliatory in their arguments towards the position of the RED method in analytical psychology.
2 Grounding a central concept of Lowen's Bioenergetic Analysis (a form of body psychotherapy) which involves the notion that the legs originate not only physical sensations but also feelings. Lively strong legs, filled with energy and planted on the ground, reflect a good perception of oneself and of external reality that results in the feeling of security and are the biologic basis for the perception of oneself as an autonomous being, capable of self-regulation. This was an invaluable discovery that Lowen brought to the world of body psychotherapy (Lowen, 1975, p. 302).
3 Procedural-associative memories of actual physical experiences.
4 In a particular instance, patients recline in a star pattern and engage in relaxation. One of them is encouraged to describe an image, and after he or she does so, another patient is urged to produce the same image. There follows a series of imagined explorations in which the two patients, one leading the way, report on their experiences and images while the rest of the group empathises. The therapist occasionally intercedes, suggesting further exploration of the sights described, or that the two patients imagine that they are joining hands and move together into a new area in the fantasised landscape. Rigo takes into account typological differences along Jungian lines, as well as being sensitive to transference issues in the course of his work. For Rigo, some of the fundamental symbolism, which is shared collectively, allows for a greater rapport between the patients who "journey" together in imagery (Rigo, 1970).

Jung and Desoille – a historical investigation

Part II

Jung and Desoille – a historical investigation

Chapter 6

Theoretical influences on Jung and Desoille

Both Jung and Desoille were influenced by spirtistic and occult practice, as well as psychical and metapsychical research. In fact, both Jung and Desoille's psychological work co-incided with the moving away of psychology from psychic research and occult phenomena to a more empirical science. They both mention that their ideas were influenced by the psychic researcher Theodore Flouroy's accounts on Helen Smith who had medium abilities, in his 1899, best-seller *Des Indes à la planète Mars : étude sur un cas de somnambulisme avec glossolalie* (Desoille, 1938; Jung, 1963/1995).

The Swiss psychologist, Theodor Flournoy, discredited the claims of spiritualists and occultists by offering a psychological explanation for the somnambulistic experiences of the medium, Helene. The book made a great impression on Jung who wrote to Flournoy volunteering to translate it. This in turn influenced Jung's 1902 research thesis on his cousin Helene Presiwerk entitled *On the Psychology and Pathology of So-Called Occult Phenomena*. Clearly, the "so-called occult" in the title of Jung's dissertation was derived from Flournoy's work and suggests that there are psychological explanations to the phenomena, not simply occult ones. Through his mother's family, Jung was part of a group in Basel involved in spiritism and séances. In his autobiography, Jung tells of the psychic happenings he experienced as a boy, and the ghost and folk stories he had heard. During his student and university years, Jung devoted a lot of time to readings on the occult and the paranormal. After finding a book on spiritism during his first year in college, Jung went on to read all of the literature on the occult available at the time. In *Memories, Dreams, Reflections*, Jung (1963) mentions books on the paranormal in the German Romantic literature of the time and mentions studies by Kerner, Swedenborg, Kant and Schopenhauer.

Desoille was a good friend of the Swiss psychologist, Pierre Bovet (Desoille, 1938) and the Swiss educator, Adolphe Ferriere (Fabre, 2014), who were colleagues of Theodore Flournoy at the "Jean Jacques Rousseau Institute" in Geneva. Flournoy[1] knew well both Bovet and Ferriere. Desoille was influenced by the French occultist Eugene Caslant born in Nanteuil-le-Haudouin, near Senlis (1865–1940) whom he met in 1923.

Desoille adapted his occultist method aimed to enhance mind reading, telepathy and clairvoyance to psychotherapy (Desoille, 1938). A footnote of the French psychologist Renaud Evrard's book, *"La légende de l'esprit: enquête sur 150 ans de parapsychology*/The Legend of the Spirit: An Inquiry into 150 Years of Parapsychology,"[2] reads:

> *Il reste encore à analyser en profondeur en quoi le "rêve éveillé dirigé" ou "onirothérapie" est d'abord une application de la métapsychique dans le champ des psychotherapies.*
>
> One still has to analyse in more depth how the waking dream method or oneirotherapy is first and foremost an application of metapsychic in the field of psychotherapy.
>
> (Evrard, 2016, p. 334 [my translation])

This link has been made only very superficially by post-Desoillians who seem to focus more on the later period of Desoille's life. In fact, Desoille referred to Caslant as *"un 'virtuose' du maniement de l'image*/a master handler of images" (Malan, 1975). Ironically, Caslant (1927/1937) used the term "passive imagination" to access these supranormal abilities and he referred to active imagination as that which is used to carry out a goal, such as writing a book. Furthermore, Desoille published three articles in the journal *Revue Metapschique* (1928, 1930 and 1932) of the *"Institut Metapsychique International*/International Metapsychic Institute" (I.M.I.) which took over from the *"Institut General Psychologique*/Institute of General Psychology," formerly *"Institut Psychologique International*/International Psychology Institute" (1900–1902). Robert Desoille and his younger brother, Henri, were very close to *Institut Metapsychique International*. Henri Desoille was a treasurer of I.M.I. in 1938 before becoming a part of the *Comité d'honneur* of I.M.I. Desoille's writings were about the psychological effects of peyote (Contribution *a l'etude des effets psychologiques du Peyotl* – Jan.—Feb. 1928), about hypnosis (*A propos de l'hypnotisme* – Nov.–Dec. 1930) and on some conditions which are needed for the success of telepathy (*De quelques conditions auxqelles il faut satisfaire pour réussir des expériences de Telephatie provoquée* – Nov.–Dec. 1932).

Desoille also presented at the third International Congress of Psychic research held at the Sorbonne in Paris in 1927. He presented a paper titled *"Un lien existe-t-il entre les états de conscience et les phénomènes électro-magnétiques?*/Is there a link between states of consciousness and electro-magnetic phenomena?" (Desoille, 1928). Jung, together with Claparede, was part of the organising committee of this congress, though Jung himself did not present at that congress (Desoille, 1928). Desoille seems to have kept his focus on researching the scientific evidence for telepathy and clairvoyance and tried to veer away from any association with the occult.

Desoille had met several occultists for research purposes and in an undated letter to Ferriere (copies found with the correspondence of Ferriere to Desoille at the Archives of the Jean Jacques Rousseau Institute), Desoille laments that Eugene Osty did not allow him to meet the famous occultist, Rudi Schneider, who was in Paris. The French author and intellectual, Rene Guenon (1971) in Vol. 1 of *Études sur la Franc-Maçonnerie et le Compagnonnage*, described one incident where a particular person tried to join a secret occult society and when asked for the password he gave them the name of M. Robert Desoille, which they had never heard of. He gave them another name unknown to them soon thereafter:

> *un certain jour, un personnage d'aspect fort louche se présenta chez nous sous prétexte de demander un emploi de secrétaire, se disant envoyé « par un de nos amis »; comme nous insistions pour savoir le nom de cet « ami », il prononça celui de M. Desoille, que nous ignorions totalement; puis, devant notre étonnement, il en donna encore un autre qui ne nous était pas moins inconnu; nous nous empressâmes naturellement d'éconduire l'individu, mais nous n'oubliâmes jamais le nom de M. Desoille.*

> One day, a person with a strong personality came to us to ask for a job of a secretary, since he was sent to us by 'one of our friends;' since we insisted on the name of this 'friend' he pronounced the name Mr. Desoille which we were ignorant of totally; then to our astonishment he gave us another name whom we never heard of before; we naturally tried to forget the episode but we never forgot the name of Mr. Desoille.
> (Gueneon, 1971, p. 183 [my translation])

Guennon adds that Desoille seemed to have heard of this incident where his name was used but insisted, in a correspondence with Dr. G. Mariani, that his interest is only *"de sujet touchant à la physique et à la psychologie/* of subject related to the physical and the psychological" (ibid., p. 183). Evidence of his scientific interest can be found in an article he wrote with Prof. Maurice Delaville in 1929, which he sent to the Academy of Science in Paris entitled *"Le métabolisme de base tel qu'il a été défini par Magnus-Lévy représente-t-il vraiment la dépense minima d'entretien de l'organisme?/* Does basal metabolism as defined by Magnus- Lévy represent the minimum expenditure of the organism?"[3] It was sent to the Academy on February 11, 1929, and he wrote again to the board of the academy to give permission to open the document on November 1, 1930. On contacting the archival department of the Academy, I was told that the letter sent to the Academy as well as the envelope have been found (in the archives of the Academy) but the article itself has been lost. Desoille makes reference to this article and his findings in his 1938 book.

Academic psychology and psychic research part company

The Fourth Congress of International Psychology, held in Paris in 1900, marked the moving away of psychology from interest in psychic research and occult phenomena. Montoro, Tortosa, Carpintiero and Piero write that there were "a large number of spiritualists, theosophists, occultists, and people interested in psychic research" (Montoro et al., 1984, p. 246) in this congress. It resulted in friction and animosity between occultists and experimental psychologists sparked by Oscar Vogt's paper "*Contre le spiritisme*/Against spiritism." In the face of such opposition, there was a sharp decline in reports by proponents of psychical research at the ensuing international congresses of psychology. Given his studies of psychological automatism in mediums and somnambules, renowned French psychiatrist, Dr. Pierre Janet, was also initially interested in the development of a centre, which carried out formal research on parapsychology. In fact, an "International Psychological Institute" was established in 1900 for the scientific study of psychical phenomena. However, when it became clear to Janet that any such study would be dominated by the parallel preoccupations of spiritualists, on the one hand, and the physical sciences, on the other, he departed. Janet's defection from the institute was sparked primarily by his desire to make of mediumship an object of psychological study and not a set of facts to be proven or disproven. Furthermore, he did not want to risk tainting his reputation when he was waiting to take over the chair of the *College de France* from Theodule Ribot (Brower, 2010, p. 56). With Janet's effective departure, the institute was legally reconstituted in 1902 as the *Institut General Psychologique* (I.G.P.). This later continued as the *Institut Metapsychique International* (I.M.I.) in Paris in 1919.

C.G. Jung Institute, metapsychic[4] research and the international metapsychical institute

Ellenberger (1970) states: "The history of the *Institut General Psychologique* has never been written, it would be interesting to know why it did not develop further and disappeared a few years later" (p. 343). M. Brady Brower (2010) continues where Ellenberger left off and gives a good account of the *Institut General Psychologique* as well as the *Institut Metapsychique Internationale*. Drawing its support from individuals with clear ties to the world of spiritism, the institute enjoyed the financial stability and social prestige that came with it. However, it also compromised its independence and raised doubts about its ability to provide the transparency necessary to carry out its research on mediumship. These doubts plagued the young institute as it set out in 1920 to provide conclusive evidence of the more extraordinary phenomena of mediumship. Following the field of psychology in its rejection of all things related to hypnotism, hysteria and unconscious mental processes, the *Institut Metapsychique Internationale* tried to stake its legitimacy on the objective method of experimental science, which in this context meant that it would stake its efforts on the materiality of mediumistic phenomena. In 1928, the *Institut Metapsychique Internationale* also piloted the idea of having a permanent congress centre in Geneva. The May–June edition of *Revue Metapsychique* of 1928 featured an article on the "Création à Genève d'un Centre Permanent de Conférences et de Congrès Internationaux de Recherches Psychiques," and names Baudouin, Ciraolo, Claparède, Driesch, Ferrière, Grandjean, Jung, Lodge, Osty, Pittard, Richet and Santoliquido at the *"Première réunion à Genève du Comité provisoire du Centre permanent de conférences et de congrès internationaux de recherches psychiques/*The first re-union in Geneva of the provisional committee of the permanent centre of international conferences and congresses on psychic research" (May–June, 1928, pp. 175–178). However, this project failed to materialise, since the idea of splitting the international psychical organisations did not go well with the "British Society of Psychic Research" (La Chapelle, 2011, p. 140).

It is in this background that we have to see Jung's contribution with an article *"La Structure de l'Ame/*The structure of the Soul" to the *Revue Metapsychique* as late as 1928. The article is a write-up of a presentation for a conference entitled *"Die Erdbedingtheit der Psyche/*The Earth's Conditioning of the Psyche," given at the "School of Wisdom" in Darmstadt in 1927 (Serina, 2013, p. 178) and published in several versions and languages and finally in French in the 1928 November–December issue of the *Revue Metapsychique*. Jung synthesises his thought at a critical turning point in his oeuvre, a moment when he abandons his work on *The Red Book* (2009) and delved into the study of alchemy (Shamdasani, 2009). Indeed, we find in Jung's text a presentation to a general audience of the fundamentals of his thought and its differences from that of Freud (Martin-Vallas, 2013). Furthermore, in the 1931 edition and the 1932 edition of the *Revue Metapsychique*, two reviews on Jung's books translated in French appear: *"Metamporphoses et symboles de la libido/*Symbols of Transformation" and *"La theorie psychoanalytique/*The Theory of Psychoanalysis."

It therefore seems that Jung, in contrast to Pierre Janet, did not mind publishing an article in a journal which did not seem to be psychologically rigorous during a period when psychology had moved its focus away from the investigation and research onto spiritistic phenomena. Nonetheless, according to the French research scholar Florent Serina (2013), Jung did not identify with the metapsychic research movement. In the E.T.H. archives, there are two letters that show that Jung had subscribed to the *Revue Metapsychique* in 1924, but there is no clue whether he continued this subscription (Serina, 2013, p. 187). Serina adds that Jung was minimally interested in the works of the members of the I.M.I. He did own several works of

Dr. Gustave Geley (1868–1924) who was the director of I.M.I. until 1924 and he references him occasionally in his works.[5] Two English translations of the works of Eugene Osty, the director who succeeded Dr. Geley at the I.M.I., can also be found in Jung's library (Serina, 2013, p. 188).

Furthermore, according to Lachapelle (2011, p. 143), French metaspychists became more critical of the academy for their inflexibility and their refusal to consider unconventional approaches and theories. The trend was towards a more mystical metapsychics and the mysteries of the Orient. Likewise, Jung also seemed to become more accepting, with the passing of time, of different explanations of psychic phenomena, other than only those of psychology. Early in his career, he tried to interpret psychic phenomena associated with spiritualism as a form of unconscious projections. However, in 1948 Jung added a footnote to his lecture "The Psychological Foundations of the Belief in Spirits," explaining that he no longer felt as certain as he did in 1919, when he had given it to the "Society for Psychical Research" (S.P.R.) that apparitions were explicable through psychology. Furthermore, in a letter of July 10, 1946 to the psychotherapist Fritz Kunkel, Jung admitted: "Metapsychic phenomena could be explained better by the hypothesis of spirits than by the qualities and peculiarities of the unconscious" (Jung, 1973, pp. 430–434).

The influence of Pierre Janet and Henri Bergson on Jung and Desoille

Both Jung and Desoille were influenced by main French thinkers such as Pierre Janet and Henri Bergson. Although Jung's French influence prior to Freud's influence on Jung has been acknowledged, there has been very little written about it (Haule, 1984; Hartman, 1994; Shamdasani, 2003). The explanation for this lies in the overwhelming success of psychoanalysis, as a result of which the earlier French psychologists have been largely forgotten (Haule, 1984). Shortly after Jung completed his medical thesis, he was given a four-month sabbatical by Bleuler in the winter of 1902–1903 during which he went to Paris to attend Janet's lectures and to meet with Binet. The period he spent in Paris to study with Janet during the winter semester of 1902–1903 is not mentioned in his autobiography (Ellenberger, 1970, p. 667). It appears that Bleuler hoped to establish some sort of a Zürich-Paris axis, involving Janet, perhaps, and engaging Binet in replications of the word association experiments being conducted in Zürich (McLynn, 1996). Since Jung was a dissociationist, his thinking followed the tradition of the French doctors Mesmer, Puysegur, Azam, Binet, Flournoy and Janet. For Janet, the unconscious consisted of one or more sub-personalities, images or ideas. His term "partial automatism" denoted a part of the person which is "split off from the awareness of the personality and which follows an autonomous, sub-conscious development" (Ellenberger, 1970,

p. 359). These split-off parts were called "subconscious fixed ideas" and feature in Jung's (1902) first major work, *On the Psychology and Pathology of So-Called Occult Phenomena*. Jung followed other researchers who studied famous mediums like Friedericke Hauffe, known as Kerner's "Seeress of Prevorst," or Charcot's Blanche Wittman (Ellenberger, 1970). Ms. "S.W.," of which later research, mainly by Charet (1993), identified her with Jung's teenage cousin Helen Preiswerk, and provided Jung with an excellent case study of somnambulistic phenomena. The most striking of these was the somnambulic character, "Ivenes," a more mature, sophisticated and socialised aspect of "S.W." (Hartmann, 1994). It is because of "Ivenes" and similar sub-personalities that Jung connects the phenomena of double consciousness to the teleological aspect of the personality which is unfolding. Jung had been stimulated enough by Janet's weekly two-hour lectures, on the impact of emotions on fluctuations in the mental level to return to Burghölzi "full of talk about Janet and his theories" (Brome, 1978, p. 83). Janet influenced Jung through his classification of the basic form of mental disease, his focus on dual personality and fixed obsessive ideas and his appreciation for neurotic patients' need to let go and sink into the subconscious. Jung also states that "My own course of development was influenced primarily by the French school and later by Wundt's psychology. Later, in 1906, I made contact with Freud, only to part company with him in 1913" (Jung, 1935, p. 773 [CW18, para.1737]).

Desoille (1938) was clearly influenced by the psychiatrist Pierre Janet, and by Sigmund Freud, as is evident in his first major book *Exploration de l'Affectivite' Subconsciente par la Méthode du Rêve Éveillé* and his articles of the 1920s. Desoille developed hypnosis into the waking dream method and he realised that he could get to the subconscious fixed ideas through the imaginative experiences of the waking dream itself. Desoille also borrowed Janet's conception of psychic energy referred as *"tension psychologique."*

Both Jung and Desoille also make reference to the French philosopher Henri Bergson (1859–1941) in their work. They make reference to his concept of *élan vital* and the creative impulse in mankind. Bergson was also involved in psychic research circles, and in 1913, he was elected as President of the "British Society of Psychical Research" (Barnard, 2012). I have found no evidence to suggest that Bergson had actually met Jung or Desoille. Bergson became a close friend of William James as can be seen from James' letters (James, 1920), who was, in turn, very close to Jung himself (Jung, 1963). According to the C.G. *Jung Bibliothek katalog* (1967), Jung kept two copies of Bergson's works in his library: *"Schopferische Entwicklung/* The creative evolution" (1912) and *"Die seelische energie/*Mind-Energy" (1928). Desoille also mentions Bergson's (1932) book *"Les Deux Sources de la Morale et de la Religion/*The Two Sources of Morality and Religion" in his 1945 book *Le Rêve Éveillé en Psychotherapie*, when he speaks of how sublimation leads to a release of creative energy. Desoille also quoted considerably in his first two books the works of another French philosopher Louis Lavelle who was also influenced by Bergson's work.

Notes

1 Flournoy died in 1920 when Desoille was 30 years old so it is unlikely that they knew each other.
2 Dr. Evrard sent me the above quote from his forthcoming book, at the time, on November 24, 2014.
3 The article is cited in *Comptes rendus des séances de l'academie des sciences – Juillet – Decembre 1930* (p. 906).
4 The term metapsychic or *metapsychique* in French should not be confused with metaphysical. It was coined by the French physiologist Charles Richet (1850–1935) in 1905. In Richet's *Traite de metapsychique*, the term is designated as "a science that has as its subject mechanical or psychological phenomena caused by forces that seem intelligent or by unknown latent powers of the human mind" (Richet, 1922, p. 5).
5 Jung's works which cite the contributions of Dr. Geley are (Jung, 1929 [1994], n. 3, p. 76; 1928–1930 [1983], p. 175; 1934–1939 [1989], pp. 449–450), and in a letter to Dr. L.M. Boyers dated September 30, 1932 (Jung, 1906–40, p. 144).

Chapter 7

Jung and Desoille

Sharing common colleagues

Jung and Desoille were born around the same time in continental Europe and both lived in small families with quite similar family compositions.[1] Yet they lived in different countries. Desoille lived in Paris for most of his life while Jung lived in Zurich, though both visited each other's country.[2]

The proximity of France to Switzerland led the two men to share several common teachers, friends and acquaintances who helped shape and develop their ideas and methods. In fact, Carl Jung developed active imagination in 1912 when he had broken his relationship with Freud, a bit before the commencement of the First World War, while Robert Desoille developed his directed waking dream method independently from Jung around 1921, a few years after the end of the same war:

> *La technique du rêve éveillé dirigé a été elaborée independamment des idees de C.G. Jung don't je n'ai connu les travaux que longtemps après le debut de mes recherché.*
>
> The directed waking dream technique was elaborated independently of the ideas of C. G. Jung, I came to know his work much later and after I had already began my research.
>
> (Desoille, 1945, p. 3 [my translation])

Common colleagues and acquaintances

Carl Jung and Robert Desoille shared common colleagues and acquaintances like Dr. Charles Baudouin the psychoanalyst from Geneva, the Swiss Doctor Joseph Marc Narcisse Guillerey, the Romanian philosopher Mircea Eliade and the Italian psychiatrist Dr. Roberto Assagioli.

Charles Baudouin (1893–1963)

Charles Baudouin was a French-Swiss psychoanalyst. He was born in Nancy, France. In his work, he combined Freud's ideas with those of Carl Jung and Alfred Adler. He lived in Geneva and founded the "Institute for

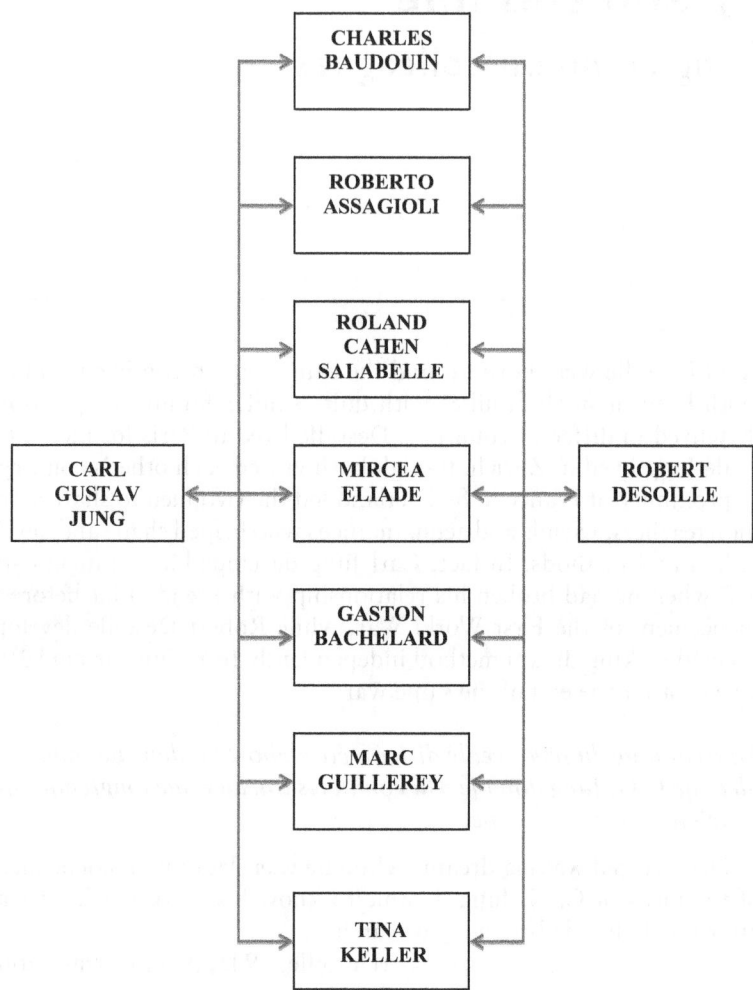

Figure 7.1 Common colleagues of Jung and Desoille.

Psychagogy and Psychotherapy" in 1924 under the patronage of Adler, Allendy, Bachelard, Besse, Coue, Driesch, Durand, Eliade, Flouroy, Flugel, Freud, Guitton, Hesnard, Hughes, Janet, Jung, Laforgue, Maeder and Meng. Later the Institute was renamed as the "International Institute for Psychoanalysis and Psychotherapy – Charles Baudouin" and is still in existence today. Dr. Baudouin knew both Desoille and Jung personally.

Dr. Baudouin was introduced to Desoille via Pierre Bovet of the "Jean Jacques Rousseau Institute" in Geneva as Baudouin himself mentions in the preface to Desoille's 1938 book. Bovet was in correspondence with

Baudouin on January 10, 1936 (Ms. fr 5954 f 6). Dr. Bovet is also mentioned as a peer researcher with Desoille in a letter to Desoille from Dr. Marc Guillery director of *La Metairie* Clinic in Nyon in Switzerland on April 30, 1935:

> *Je suis tres interesse par les recherché que vous avez entrepresies avec Monsieur Bovet et me rejouis de connaire vos observations*
>   I am very interested in the research that you have undertaken with Mr Bovet and would love to know about your findings.
>   (Malan, 1975, p. 19)

Baudouin had invited Desoille to write in his journal as early as the 1920s. Desoille did take up the offer with a number of his articles appearing over the years in *Action et Pensée* (14 articles from 1931 to 1963). Baudouin puts Desoille's research in relation to Jung's, and points out that Desoille's method can appear "as a systematic development of the sessions of Jung's active imagination" (Baudouin, 1950/2007, p. 70).

Baudouin, who incidentally shared the same birthday as Jung, had been in correspondence with Jung from the early 1920s. The 29 letters between Baudouin and Jung found at the E.T.H. library in Zurich are dated between 1924 and 1955. Baudouin published several articles on analytical psychology in the journal *Action et Pensée* and in 1963, he published a book on Jung's work and analytical psychology, "*L'Oeuvre de Jung et la Psychologie Complexe*/The Work of Jung and Complex Psychology," making it one of the earliest biographies of Jung. Baudouin had also invited Jung to submit an article for the journal *Action et Pensée*. As a result, Jung published three articles on "Psychological types" in Baudouin's journal. Jung's articles appeared in the January, February and March editions of 1931. The article entitled "*Seelenprobleme der Gegenwart*/The Soul Problem in Modern Times" was published in April 1933 (No. 4) while the article "*L'expérience des associations*/The Association Experiences" was in the February edition of 1944 (no. 2). The latter does not appear in Jung's *Collected Works*. In a letter from Baudouin to Jung dated October 14, 1930 (HS 1056: 542), Baudouin thanks Jung for sending a copy of one of his works and asks Jung for permission to reprint some of the material in *Action et Pensée* (this seems to refer to Jung's articles appearing in the 1931 editions of *Action et Pensée*). Jung gives his permission in a letter to Baudouin dated October 20, 1930 (Hs 1056: 658). Incidentally, Desoille contributed to the May edition of 1931 with an article titled "Une méthode rationnelle pour l'exploration du subconscient." Dr. Richard Bevand,[3] a disciple of Desoille who also served as the secretary of Charles Baudouin, was also introduced to Jung by Baudouin (Bevand, personal communication).[4] He told me that copies of the journal *Action et Pensée* must have been sent to Jung. In Jung's library in Kusnacht, there are 11 volumes of the collection *Action et Pensée* dated between 1943 and 1947, some of them have been used, some have not been

(Andreas Jung, personal communication).[5] A number of these copies are dedicated to Jung. The September 1955 (no. 3) special edition of the journal *Action et Pensée* is a "*Hommage à Jung à l'occasion de son 80ème anniversaire*/Homage to Jung on the Occasion of his 80th Birthday." A copy of it is found in the Separata section of the E.T.H. library. Dr. Richard Bevand, in a letter to Jung dated May 16, 1955, asks him for his portrait to be included in this special edition (HS 1056: 21'028). Furthermore, in a letter dated January 5, 1958, Dr. Bevand offers Jung, as an honorary member, a free subscription to the revue *Action et Pensée* (HS 1056: 21'216). Jung was an honorary member of the "*Société de Psychagogie et de Psychothérapie*/Society of Psychology and Psychotherapy" as shown in the letter that Baudouin sent to Jung on April 9, 1925 (HS 1056: 98). If Jung had received copies of the *Revue Action et Pensée* from the 1930s, especially those published in 1931, he could have heard about Desoille and his work from as early as 1931. However, these editions prior to 1943 could not be traced. In a letter dated November 17, 1928 (HS 1056: 210), Baudouin also asks Jung if he would be able to teach in Geneva on May 13, 1929. Jung also kept five books written by Baudouin. In at least one of them "*De l'Instinct a l'Esprit*/From Instinct to Spirit" (1950), he makes five different citations on Desoille and his method.

Another valuable clue about Jung and Desoille's connection comes via Tina Keller[6] from Geneva. Tina Keller was initially analysed by Jung, Toni Wolf and Baudouin[7] (Swan, 2007). She also wrote an article on active imagination in 1941, entitled "L'imagination active," where she mentions both Jung's active imagination and Robert Desoille's directed waking dream method. Keller also mentions Desoille's 1938 book in her 1940 book, "*L'Ame et le Nerfs*/The Soul and Nerves" (PP/TKR/7), which Charles Baudouin helped her publish: "Professor Charles Baudouin, who was an experienced writer, out of friendship helped me organise the book and he also wrote the preface." She writes that "*Desoille de Paris a publie un livre sur 'le rêve éveillé' qui est analogue a 'l'imagination active*/Desoille from Paris has published a book on the 'waking dream' which is similar to active imagination" (Keller, 1941, p. 176). Tina Keller remained in correspondence with Charles Baudouin between August 1923 and April 29, 1963 (seven letters available at the archives of the *Bibliotheque nationale de Geneve, Charles Baudouin Papers Collection*).

Joseph Marc Narcisse Guillerey (1895–1954)

In Romandy, Switzerland, Dr. Marc Guillerey was the main pioneer in the psychotherapeutic use of guided imaginative therapeutic techniques. He began his experiments with the method as early as 1925. He officially named the method "*rêverie dirigé*/guided reverie" in 1942 but later changed the name to "*rêve vecu*/ experiential dream," allowing more spontaneous expression rather than a directive approach. Unfortunately, he never published the manuscript he worked on during his life and thus remains an unknown figure in the history of mental imagery (Guggisberg, 1995, p. 213). His theoretical orientation was rooted in psychosomatic concepts which were in part derived from his association with the Lausanne physician, Roger Vittoz[8] (Vittoz, 1911/1937). In his emphasis on the importance of being immersed in the imaginal body, Guillerey prefigures the work of Dr. Andre Virel (Virel & Fretigny, 1968), who also believes that the success of his "oneirotherapeutic" method is in large measure a result of the degree to which the subject is fully in his imaginal body during the imagery session. Guillerey worked in Nyon in the Metairie clinic, spent some time in Vevey and later settled in Lausanne (Guggisberg, 1995).

Dr. Guillerey was one of Desoille's early disciples in the 1930s. Guggisberg mentions that in the minutes of February 9, 1935 of the study group founded by Pere Amiable and Robert Desoille, there were *"members des religieux, des laics et des medecins don't Guillerey, d'Espiney, Pourtal, entre autres*/religious members, lay persons and doctors such as Guillerey, d'Espiney, Pourtal, amongst others" (Guggisberg, 1995, p. 229 [my translation]). Charles Baudouin also mentions Dr. Guillerey in the preface to Desoille's *Exploration de l'Affectivité Subconsciente par la Méthode du Rêve Eveillé: Sublimation et Acquisitions Psychologiques* and how his efforts have concluded important results (Desoille, 1938).

There is a correspondence between Dr. Guillerey and Desoille from 1934 to 1937 which is cited in an article by Sivadon (1967) and in Malan's thesis (1975). At one point, the relationship between Desoille and Guillerey was somewhat broken since Dr. Guillerey was implying that he had discovered his method of *rêve dirigé* independently of Desoille. Guggisberg mentions that Dr. Guillerey was impressed by seeing Pere Amiable, another colleague of Desoille's, perform a session on a person in Switzerland. Nonetheless, they did make up in the end as can be seen from the article *"Notes sur le pouvoir regenerateur du 'rêve dirigé'*/Notes on the regenerating power of the directed dream," written by Charles Baudouin as a homage to Guillerey in *Action et Pensée* of December 1954 after Dr. Guillerey's death at the young age of 59. In it, Baudouin explains that Guillerey was influenced by *"la psychoanalyse, la mtéhode de Desoille, les exercises de Loyola/* psychoanalysis, the method of Desoille, the exercises of Loyola" (Baudouin, 1954, p. 114). Guillerey was friends with Claperede, Oscar Forel, Piaget, Baudouin and Bachelard, and was analysed by Dr. Henri Flournoy. Guggisberg (1995) also claims that Dr. Guillerey knew Jung. Guggisberg's claims were personally confirmed by Guillerey's grandson Cyril Baechtold-Guillerey.[9] The latter added that Guillerey used to attend Jung's conferences in Zurich. Moreover, at the E.T.H. library, in Jung's collection of offprints/special prints, I found an offprint of Guillerey's article *"Une nouvelle méthode psychothérapique*/A new method of psychotherapy," edited by Jacques Mai, which was published in *Psyché* No. 105-106. It includes neither the place nor the year of publication.

This refers to the journal *Psyche* of 1955 (No. 10: 105), which featured the paper read at a conference held in 1942. Guggisberg mentions that Guillerey corresponded with Jung on a patient's artwork with the name of Stella, who later continued to practise his method: "*Il resort des notes personenelles de Guillerey que ce dernier (Stella) a eu un echange avec Jung au sujet des productions de cette malade*/From Guillerey's private notes emerges that Stella's work was the subject of an exchange with Jung" (Guggisberg, 1995, p. 233). Unfortunately, this correspondence between Jung and Guillerey was not found at the E.T.H. library. After Guillerey's death, the family gave the paintings to Jean Dubuffet. However, when I contacted the Jean Dubuffet museum in Lausanne, the paintings could not be traced (personal electronic communication by curator Pascale Marini-Jeanneret dated August 13, 2015). Furthermore, Guggisberg describes how the Jesuit Pere de Chambost has written an article[10] where he states the Zurich professor (C.G. Jung) had publicly shown his personal admiration for Guillerey (ibid., p. 233). Despite such a strong statement, Jung does not mention Guillerey in any of his works, even though one has to keep in mind that in the late 40s and 50s when Guillerey's method was well developed, Jung was well advanced in age.

Mircea Eliade (1907–1986)

Mircea Eliade, a Romanian philosopher and historian of religion, had met Desoille in 1945 after the death of his first wife Lucie. He knew of his psychological writings involving inner imaginative movement along a vertical axis. Mircea Eliade wrote about myths and symbols in his works (1951, 1952, 1959). In his *Journal I*, Eliade wrote that Desoille used the:

> symbols, myths and rituals which I myself discussed in 'Le Probleme du chamanisme.' Thus he has cured neuroses and other kind of mental illness by using (without knowing) elements of shamanistic rituals and symbols of ascension (which as I have shown in my study, are something entirely different from 'primitive magical practises.'
>
> (Eliade, 1973, p. 40)

This affirms Desoille's interest in the symbolic and its curative value. In 1947, in a volume in honour of the great art historian, Ananda K. Coomarswamy, Eliade dedicated an article to the symbolic *Durohana*, a term that indicates the "difficult path" which is linked to India's Vedic rituals and shamanic practices of ascension. Eliade mentioned this aspect in relation to a specific phase of Desoille's method based on the *rêve éveillé*, and noted how the therapeutic process based on inviting patients to imagine a "climbing dream" by climbing either a ladder or a mountain resulted in a "complete recovery, even in serious cases where previous psychoanalytical treatment had not brought the slightest improvement"

(Eliade, 1947, p. 209). Eliade inferred that "through the repetition of an archetypical gesture the psyche recovers its integrity and regains its lost structural unity" and explained this as a "spiritual technique applied to psychical fact" (ibid., pp. 209–210).

According to Oldmeadow (1995), Eliade was definitely in correspondence with Jung between 1948 and 1955, as shown in the E.T.H. archives and they had also met several times at Eranos. Eliade was first invited to the annual Eranos conferences in 1950 and attended annually until 1962, the year of Olga Froebe's death, delivering lectures at most conferences. In his *Journal I*, Eliade, on August 23, 1950, recounts his first meeting with Jung at a dinner at a restaurant in Ancona:

> he is a captivating old gentleman, utterly without conceit, who is as happy to talk as he is to listen. What could I write down here first of this long conversation? Perhaps his bitter reproaches of 'official science'? In university circles he is not taken seriously.
>
> (Eliade cited in Wehr, 1988, pp. 273–274)

In an interview late in his life, Eliade again recalled his first meeting with Jung:

> After half an hour's conversation I felt I was listening to a Chinese sage or an east European peasant, still rooted in the Earth Mother yet close to Heaven at the same time. I was enthralled by the wonderful simplicity of his presence [...].
>
> (Eliade, 1982, pp. 162–163)

In 1952, Eliade conducted a lengthy interview with Jung for the Parisian magazine *Combat: de la Resistance a la Revolution*, which was published on October 9, 1952, at a time when Jung's recently published *Answer to Job* was provoking a stormy controversy (Eliade, 1952/1977, p. 225). In the same year, Jung read Eliade's work on shamanism and the two had a long discussion about it. They met several times over the next few years, the last occasion being at Kusnacht in 1959 where they had a lengthy conversation in the garden, primarily about the nature of mystical experience (Oldmeadow, 1995).

Eliade's relationship with Jung[11] was stronger than that with Desoille, since as we have already mentioned, he seems to have only met Desoille once. However, Eliade seems to have been influenced in his writings by both Jung and Desoille.

Roberto Assagioli (1888–1974)

Roberto Assagioli was an Italian psychiatrist, psychoanalyst and pioneer in the fields of humanistic and transpersonal psychology. He is the founder of the therapeutic school known as Psychosynthesis. He was a friend of Carl Jung from the early years of the twentieth century and in the 1950s he became acquainted with Robert Desoille.

When I asked if there was any possible correspondence between Assagioli and Desoille or Dr. Guilhot, in the archives of Assagioli's house in Florence, no evidence emerged. However, the archives and newsletters (from 1958 to 1974) of the "Psychosynthesis Research Foundation" in America proved to be a good source of relevant information. In fact, included in the section of Psychosynthesis in Europe, in the seventh newsletter[12] of the Psychosynthesis Research Foundation issued in September 1959, Assagioli describes his meeting in Paris at Dr. Guilhot house which served as the *Centre de Psychosynthese*: "Apart from the meeting I had long and valuable conversations with Prof. Baruk, Mr. Desoille and Dr. J. Lepp" (p. 3). Further proof that Assagioli knew Desoille comes from the French psychoanalyst Madame Nicole Fabre (2002), who was analysed by Robert Desoille in the 60s. She describes how she was invited to attend a conference in Switzerland organised by Dr. Jean Guilhot. During this conference, Paul Diel, Roberto Assagioli and Robert Desoille were present (Fabre, 2002). This same conference is also described by Dr. Guilhot in the 18th edition of "*La Revue de Psychosynthese*/Review of Psychosynthesis" of February 2006, where he explains how this conference was organised in 1960 by Solange de Merignac, Marie-Aimee Guilhot and himself. The panel included "Suzanne Nouvion, Jacqueline de Chevron Villette, Ignace Lepp, Paul Diel, Charles Baudouin, Nicolas Fabre" to name a few (Guilhot, 2006, p. 7).

Desoille's disciple, Dr. Jean Guilhot, started to hold psychosynthesis meetings in his house in Paris in 1958 and became the co-ordinator of Psychosynthesis training in Paris (second newsletter, November 1958 of the "Psychosynthesis Research Foundation"). Desoille also lectured at the "Three week International conference of Psychosynthesis" held at the *Institut Le Bleu Leman*, in Villeneuve, near Montreux in Switzerland between August 24 and 31, 1960 (tenth Newsletter, July 1960 of the Psychosynthesis Research Foundation, U.S.A.). Desoille took part again in the International Conference of Psychosynthesis of 1962, where he gave a lecture entitled "Theory and practice of the *Rêve éveillé*." It is very interesting to see that at the time Desoille had embraced Pavlovian principles to explain his method. He was using the Psychosynthesis fora to present his work.

In the symposium on psychosynthesis which was held on August 24, 1961 during the fifth International Congress of Psychotherapy, organised at the University of Vienna, Dr. Robert Gerard of Los Angeles, California, presented a paper in English entitled "The Guided Daydream in Psychosynthesis." In this paper, he illustrated how the *Rêve éveillé* technique of Robert Desoille can be applied to individual and group psychosynthesis

(14th newsletter[13] of "Psychosynthesis Research Foundation," October 1961, p. 2). This shows how Desoille[14] was "adopted" by the Psychosynthesis movement and how his work was being demonstrated to a larger international audience. Desoille also took part in organising a small group of autopsychosynthesis in Paris (the 22nd February newsletter[15] issue of 1964 of "Psychosynthesis Research Foundation"):

> The pattern adopted by the meeting allowed a comparison of two methods of working on the first day as one large group; and on the second, in three sections or sub-groups. The speakers included Dr. Guilhot, Mlle. S Nouvion (Director of the Recherches et Rencontres Association), Robert Desoille, Yvonne Schlesser, Marie-Louise Collard and Dane Rudhyar.[16]
>
> (1964, p. 2)

The long-term professional and friendly relationship between Jung and Assagioli began in 1907 and lasted until Jung's death in 1961. Assagioli joined the Geneva circle of Edouard Claparede and Theodore Flournoy (Berti, 1988) in the early years of the twentieth century. His collaboration with them on the study of associations was the main reason for Assagioli's first trip to Zurich (1907), where he had his first contact with Jung. Assagioli was at that time a Freudian psychiatrist and psychoanalyst. Jung, in a letter of August 12, 1907, addressed to Freud, almost certainly referred to Assagioli when he wrote "in just three weeks seven Americans, a Russian, an Italian, and a Hungarian were here" (McGuire, 1974, p. 76).

After the Sixth International Congress of Psychology in Geneva (August 2–7, 1909), at which Assogioli joined other Italian colleagues and founded the Italian Psychological Society, he returned to work at Burghozli to draft his dissertation on psychoanalysis (Berti, 1988). Although Jung left the Burgholzli in 1909 to devote himself exclusively to his private practice in Kusnacht, Assagioli frequently visited him. The visits continued after he graduated, as Assagioli valued the depth of their conversations which took place in Jung's study and which was full of books and exotic objects (Giovetti, 1995). In a letter to Jung in January 1946, Assagioli mentioned the memorable hosting he received from Jung in 1939 when he passed through Zurich on the way to Italy (HS 1056: 12 246). In the same letter, Assagioli also asked Jung if he could help him enter Switzerland in order to accompany his son, affected by tuberculosis, to the sanatorium in Leysin (French Switzerland). Such correspondence proves that Assagioli's relationship with Jung was not only professional but also personal. I found seven letters between Jung and Assagioli at the E.T.H. archives between 1932 and 1948. Despite the lack of written evidence, their relationship lasted for a long time.

Notes

1 In fact, both Carl Gustav Jung and Robert Desoille were the eldest children in their families. Carl Jung had a younger sister, Gertrude (Bair, 2003), and Robert Desoille had a younger brother named Henri. Jung and Desoille both lost their fathers when they were 21 years old and both had mothers who exerted a great influence on them.

2 Desoille is known to have visited the French-speaking Switzerland (Romandie) as he was friend with the Swiss Dr. Marc Guillery of Nyon. Guillery formed part of Desoilles' *Circle d'etudes* in the early 1930s (Malan, 1975). Desoille was also friends with Adolphe Ferriere (AdF/C/1/18), as well as the Genevan psychoanalyst, Dr. Charles Baudouin, who allowed him to publish his work in the journal of his institute. In a letter dated October 4, 1944, Desoille writes to the Director General of *Presses Universitaires de France* how Dr. Baudouin would help mention his book, written in 1945, to the Swiss public and how he would be publishing a small booklet with Mont Blanc editors in Switzerland to engage the Swiss readers. He also visited Villeneuve, near Montreux, Switzerland, for the International Convention on Psychosynthesis in 1960.

   Jung also visited Paris on several occasions: in 1902/03 to meet with Binet and Janet, in the spring of 1907 for a meeting with Janet, in March of 1910 and in 1932 to teach seminars at *Club du Gros Caillou*. In 1932, only Jung's wife Emma gave the lecture. Jung gave a presentation in Paris on the collective unconscious in May, 1934 (Serina, 2018). One of his daughters, Gret Baumann-Jung, lived in Paris for 12 years with her family from 1926, so it is likely that Jung went to visit her. Jung's wife also spent some months in Paris just before she married Jung (Gaudissart, 2014). It is also worth noting that Jung was fluent in French.

3 Bevand passed away in January 2019.

4 Bevand corresponded with me on this issue via e-mail through his wife Ms. Kirsten Adamzik on December 26, 2012.

5 In a correspondence to me dated January 8, 2015, Mr. Andreas Jung writes: "There are 11 volumes of the 'Collection Action et Pensée' in the library dated between 1943 and 1947, some of them are used, some not. Some are dedicated to Jung."

6 Tina Keller was the wife of a close friend of Jung, Prof. Adolf Keller, who also wrote an article in the *Revue Action et Pensée* entitled "C.G. *Jung et la crise de notre temps*," in September 1955.

7 Tina Keller writes in Section E with the heading "I work as a Jungian Analyst" of a document titled "Recollections of my encounter with Dr. Jung" kept at the Archives of the Welcome Library in London, in 1941, that she "had the privilege of doing psychological work with Professor Charles Baudouin" (E-6 PP/TKR/2/1).

8 Roger Vittoz was a Swiss physician born on May 6, 1863 in Morges and died on April 10, 1925 in Lausanne. He is one of the first psychsomaticians. He developed a therapeutic method known as the Vittoz method since he was not satisfied with hypnosis. His main book was written in 1911 entitled *"Traitement des psychonévroses par la rééducation du contrôle cerebral/Psychoneurotic Treatment through the Re-Education of Cerebral Control."* With it he treated T.S. Eliot.

9 In an e-mail sent to me by Mons. Cyril Baechtold on July 28, 2015, he confirmed:

   Mon grand père a effectivement rencontré C.J.Jung ou, en tous cas assisté a des conférences et des cours donnés par Jung à Zürich/ My grand father has effectively met C. J. Jung and attended some of the conferences and courses given by Jung in Zurich.

No dates are given about when these possible meetings could have taken place.

10 The article "Un grand psychotherapeute, le Dr. Marc Guillerey" by the Jesuit Pere de Chambost S. J., who knew Dr. Guillerey, was published after Guillerey's death in the *Gazette de Lausanne* on October 16 and 17, 1954.

11 For an in-depth study of Eliade and Jung, see Dr. T. Velletri's unpublished doctoral thesis titled *Mircea Eliade and C.G. Jung: A Comparative Study*, 2015, University of Essex – Centre for Psychoanalytic Studies, U.K.

12 This letter can be accessed from the online archive of the Psychosynthesis Research Foundation, U.S.A. at www.psychosynthesisresources.com/.

13 This letter can be accessed from the same online archive of the Psychosynthesis Research Foundation.

14 Desoille's niece, Monique Pellerin (1925–2005), after Desoille's death also joined the *Institut Francais de Psychosynthese* in Paris, where she served as its second president. She also published a book entitled *La Psychosynthese* together with Micheline Bres in 1994. An article in June 2005, by Micheline Bres of *La Revue de Psychosynthese*, pays homage to her.

15 This letter can be accessed from the online archive of the Psychosynthesis Research Foundation, USA at www.psychosynthesisresources.com/.

16 Interestingly Desoille's friend, the Swiss educator Adolphe Ferriere, was a disciple of the transpersonal astrologist and composer Dane Rudhyar.

Chapter 8

Unacknowledged European imaginative therapeutic practitioners

Given the common colleagues that both Jung and Desoille shared, one may wonder if they had actually met or corresponded given the fact that Desoille did not hesitate to open his method to Jungian teachings. My research on this matter took me to the E.T.H. library in Zurich to see if there was any correspondence between the two.

The correspondence between Desoille and Jung

To my surprise, I found out that Desoille did send to Jung a signed copy of his first book *Exploration de l'Affectivité Subconsciente par la Methode du Rêve éveillé: Sublimation et Acquisitions Psychologiques* (still available intact in Jung's library, Kusnacht), possibly with a letter.[1] The note on the book says: "*Hommage de l'auteur au Doctuer C. G. Jung en temoignage de sa profonde admiration*/Homage of the author to Doctor C.G. Jung as a witness of my profound admiration."

Jung's secretary wrote a thank you letter to Desoille on March 22, 1938 (Hs 1056: 7283, see copy of letter below) stating that since Jung was indisposed for health reasons, she was replying instead of him, and thanking him for the book while hoping that he could read it when possible. This letter is proof that Jung must at least heard of Desoille. Nonetheless, nothing came out of this correspondence. For some reason, Jung did not continue to correspond with Desoille. A year later, the latter is nostalgic about this lost opportunity to engage in a correspondence with Jung. In the archives of the "Jean Jacques Rousseau Institute" in Geneva, I found a copy of correspondence between Desoille and the Swiss Adolphe Ferriere (1938–1946), besides the original letters dated 1938 sent by Ferriere to Desoille (AdF/C/1/18). In part of a letter Desoille writes to Ferriere, dated June 9, 1939, Desoille mentioned that he had read the *Secret of the Golden Flower*, of which Jung wrote the introduction. Desoille added:

> *Jung est un homme pour qui j'ai une profonde admiration; il etait malade quand il a recu mon livre et je croins qu'il ne l'ai jamais lu*
> Jung is a person I admire a lot, he was sick when he received my book and I think he has never read it.
>
> (Desoille, 1939 [my translation])

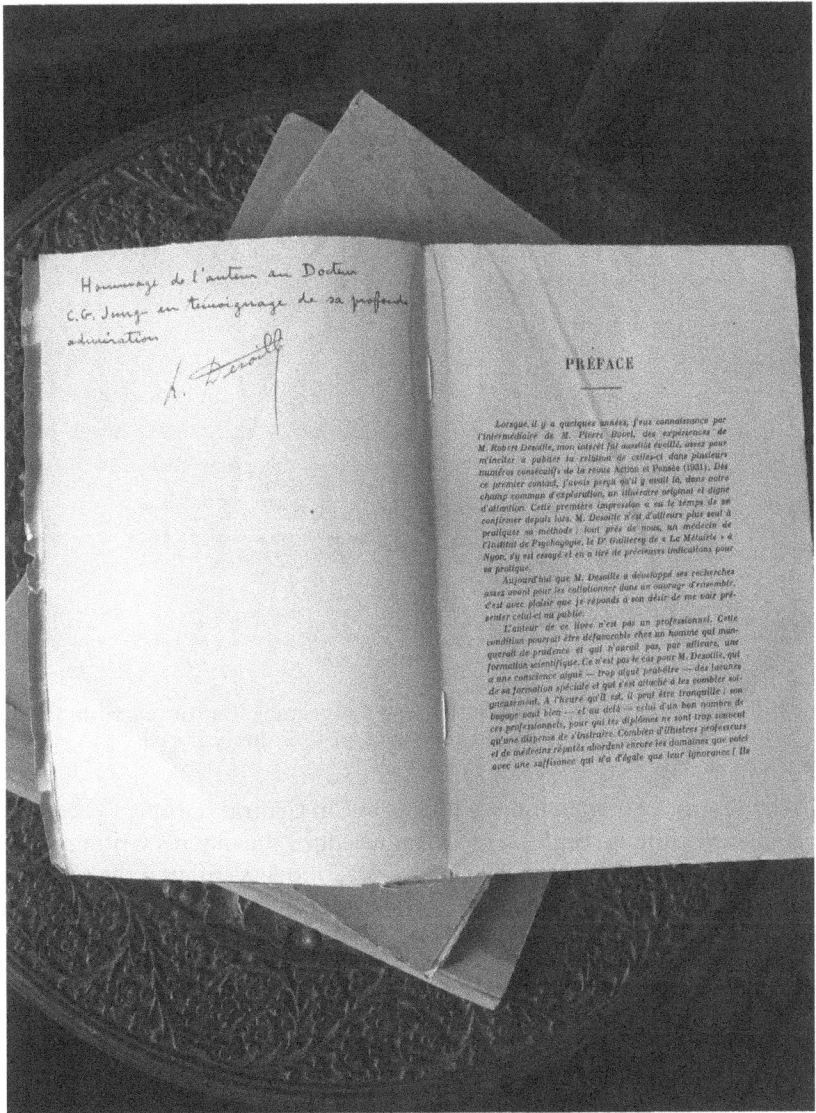

Figure 8.1 Desoille's signed book copy to Jung. Reprinted with permission of Foundation of the Works of C.G. Jung, Zurich.

Unacknowledged practitioners of waking dream methods who were in contact with Jung

Desoille was very much disappointed with Jung's brief letter via his secretary which spelled little hope for future collaboration. An almost similar fate seemed to have fallen on other practitioners who were working with

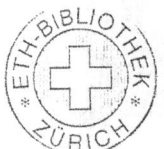

le 22 mars, 1938.

Monsieur Robert Desoille,
9 rue Falguière,
Paris XVe.

Monsieur,

Le Docteur Jung étant empêché pour cause de santé de vous écrire lui-même, me charge de vous remercier de l'aimable envoi de votre livre sur la "Méthode du rêve éveillé." Il se réjouit de le lire dès que cela lui sera possible.

Veuillez agréer, Monsieur, mes salutations distinguées.

secrétaire.

Figure 8.2 Letter sent to Desoille by Jung's secretary. Reprinted with permission of Foundation of the Works of C.G. Jung, Zurich.

different forms of imagination in Jung's time in Central Europe.[2] These were in contact with Jung, but he never acknowledged them in his writings. I will describe the possible reasons why these practitioners suffered the same fate of Desoille, i.e., not receiving any acknowledgement or referencing by Jung.

Jung and Carl Happich

Around the same time Desoille wrote to Jung, the latter was also in correspondence with Dr. Carl Happich (1878–1947), a German doctor from Darmstadt who also worked with guided imagery and guided meditation between 1933 and 1938 (E.T.H. Bibliothek, C.G. Jung Papers Collection). Dr. Happich was a friend of Count Keyserling, who was very close to Jung himself. The German Jungian analyst Gustav Heyer was also a student of Dr. Happich. Happich was a founder member of Keyserling's "School of Wisdom"[3] and was a member of the Evangelical Brotherhood of St. Michael, a German religious Brotherhood belonging to the Berneuchen Movement,[4] which formed part of the Lutheran Liturgical Movement. He developed meditative imaginative exercises for the evangelical church and became a pioneer of modern meditation.[5] According to the researcher, Prof. (Dr.) Karl Baier (2013), Happich's meditative exercises were influenced by the Viennese psychoanalyst Herbert Silberer (1882–1923) and by *The Gospel of Relaxation* of William James (1842–1910) (p. 60). This *Gospel of Relaxation* is a chapter in James' (1911) book "On Vital Reserves: The Energies of Men." Happich also carried forward the work of the French Alfred Binet of "provoked introspection," which was brought to Germany by the Wurzburg group. Moreover, Happich elaborated on Binet's early work by facilitating the emergence of images through the use of muscle relaxation and meditative states (Watkins, 1976, pp. 54–55). Happich's work became known in the Anglo-American world through the help of Wolfgang Kretschmer, son of the famous psychiatrist Ernst Kretschmer. Wolfgang was also involved with St. Michael's Brotherhood. Hanscarl Leuner, the founder of Kathymic Imaginative psychotherapy, based his method on Happich's therapeutic method after hearing one of his lectures (Baier, 2013).

My research at the E.T.H. library in Zurich found that Happich wrote to Jung on 14 May, 1934 (Hs. 1056: 2781). Happich described how he had sent Jung a copy of his article on his guided imagery method on January 10, 1933, which appeared in the *Zentralblatt fur psychotherapie* of November 1932, entitled "*Das Bildbewusstsein als ansatzstelle psychischer Behandlung*/Image consciousness as a rudimentary form of psychological treatment." Jung replied on January 16, 1933 (Hs 1056: 2421), saying that it left an "*interessanten sonderabdruckes*/special impression" on him. Nonetheless, Jung does not reference Happich in his works. There are seven letters in all between Happich and Jung, at the E.T.H. archives.

Jung and Alfred Wolfsohn

Between September 27, 1937 and February 21, 1939, Alfred Wolfsohn was in correspondence with Jung about the possibility of Jung giving his expert view on Alfred Wolfsohn's therapeutic approach using the voice[6] (Pikes, 2005). Jung kept saying he was busy until May 3, 1955, where Aniela Jaffe wrote him a letter on Jung's behalf, telling him to contact Mrs. Dora Kalf who "is keen on music and will have the necessary understanding for your work" (Pikes, 2005, pp. 172–173). Therefore, Jung was very much aware of the European imaginative psychotherapies that were being practised during his times. The focus on the imagination was still very relevant in Central Europe amongst European psychologists who seemed unperturbed by the growing emphasis of behaviourism in America. This was due to the fact that many of the experimentalists had fled Europe during the First and Second World Wars and there was a strong influence of German and French phenomenology. The latter was serving as a philosophical basis of European clinical psychology as well as the rise of translated subjective Eastern texts in Europe (Sheikh & Jordan, 1983, p. 396).

Jung's lack of acknowledgement of European imaginative psychotherapeutic practitioners

One may speculate on why Jung failed to acknowledge the above-mentioned European imaginative therapeutic practitioners of his time, who corresponded with him, besides Desoille, Guillerey and Leuner, which we have already mentioned. I will give three possible hypotheses as to why Jung failed to do so.

First of all, Jung did not make reference to other therapeutic imagery practitioners of his time, since he might have wanted to make sure to safeguard the originality of his method as distinct from other contemporary Western approaches. Jung seems to have suffered from the proverbial "anxiety of influence" (Bloom, 1973) not only from his predecessors but also from his peers. Savage (2011) has described how Jung knowingly participated in concealing and distorting important information throughout his career for his own gain. Jung's failure to acknowledge European imaginative practitioners which were in correspondence with him is another case in point.

Another possible explanation is that Jung had already moved his interest to alchemy from active imagination by 1930, and thus he might have not really been interested in referencing European practitioners who started to publish their works in the 10s, 20s and 30s. However, one also has to note that despite Jung's obsession with researching alchemy from the 1930s onwards, he still continued to mention active imagination in his works. Thus, the hypothesis of Jung choosing to focus his interest just on alchemy is not so tenable. In fact, Jung used the term "active imagination" for the first time in *The Tavistock Lectures* in 1935 since previously he had referred to his therapeutic method using different names. Furthermore, in his final work, *Mysterium Coniunctionis*, Jung (1955/1970) described active imagination as the way towards self-knowledge and individuation. It is also worth noting that Jung had commenced a comparative study of active imagination through a series of seminars at the E.T.H. University in Zurich, known as the "ETH Lectures," between 1933 and 1941. In these lectures, which have not yet been fully published, he compared active imagination to other older transformation systems of the East and the West. In fact, he compared his technique with Patanjali's Yoga sutras and Buddhist meditational practices, with "The Spiritual Exercises of Saint Ignatius of Loyola"[7] and with the meditations of alchemical philosophy, but again failed to mention other European imaginative psychotherapeutic approaches of his time. Moreover, in 1933, Jung also took part in the Conference at Eranos titled *Yoga and Meditation in East and West*. The conferences of 1936 and 1937 also had similar themes, namely the *Idea of Redemption in the East and the West*.

The last hypothesis is founded on the idea that Jung was more interested in comparing active imagination with much older and grander approaches both in the East and West, rather than with the new developing imagery approaches in the West. In fact, Jung maintained a cautious attitude towards the general interest in Oriental Yoga methods, which were spreading widely in Europe. Jung continuously criticised systems such as the theosophical ones, which in his view imitated Oriental methods and techniques of meditation. Dutch scholar, Olga Fröbe-Kapteyn, who organised the "Eranos" meetings, agreed with Jung's ideas on this matter and in her Foreword to the Yearbook, dedicated to "East-Western Symbolism and Soul Guidance" (Ostwestliche Symbolik und Seelenführung), she repeated Jung's concerns when she points out: "building the Western path to salvation must grow on Western ground, and must be elaborated with Western symbols and formed with Western material." Olga Fröbe illustrates here the presence in the Western world of a "proper Yoga tradition," namely in the "'mystical schools' of the Gnostics, Hermetics and Pythagoreans and of the later alchemical mystical Rosicrucian traditions" (Sorge, 2009, pp. 394–395). So it seems that Jung emphasised a vertical historical comparative approach to active imagination more than a horizontal, historical one which might have included the European imagery practitioners with methods heavily influenced from Eastern sources. In this way, Jung positions himself as the heir of older traditions.

Notes

1 Desoille's letter was not found but only his signed book and Jung's reply through his secretary.
2 While Jeremy Holmes (2014) describes imaginative therapeusis as an Anglo-Saxon contribution to psychoanalytic clinical theory through the influence of English Romantic writers and German philosophical Idealism on Sharpe, Bion, Winnicott and Rycroft, one also needs to mention the imaginative practitioners such as Carl Happich, Robert Desoille, Marc Guillery and Alfred Wolfsohn who pioneered imaginative therapeusis in Central Europe in the 1900s through Occult practices and Eastern meditative influences.
3 The psychoanalyst Walter Frederking who was associated with Keyserling's "School of Wisdom" developed a therapeutic method similar to that of Happich. It is possible that there may have been a direct influence from Happich himself (Baier, 2013).
4 The Berneuchen Movement is part of the Lutheran Liturgical movement in Germany. It originates from the German Youth Movement. The movement was born in the 1920s, after the radical changes caused by the First World War. The founders felt that it was necessary to give to the spiritual life a greater and more perfect concrete form, in order to throw off the influence of liberal theology. The group met annually in the Berneuchen Manor near Neudamm, which gave the name for the circle. In 1926, the circle published *Berneuchener Buch*, written by Karl Bernhard Ritter, Wilhelm Stählin, Ludwig Heitmann (de) and Wilhelm Thomas.
5 Frizo Melzer (1907–1990) continued with Happich's methods on meditation. He considered himself as the last student of Happich before Happich's death.

Similar developments were also done by the theologian Karl Bernhard Ritter, who was a friend of Happich from the Evangelical Brotherhood of St. Michael (Baier, 2013).

6 Alfred Wolfsohn sought to rid himself of terrible ongoing suffering through the use of voice. In the trenches of the First World War, he heard the terrible cries of injured and dying men. After the war he suffered from post-traumatic stress disorder which manifested in the form of aural hallucinations, replaying the agonised human sounds of the battlefield. To free himself of the voices which persecuted him, he began to emulate with his own voice the sounds he heard inside until he healed himself. Through his self-investigation, he came to understand that the human voice is the expression of the self, that one is revealed in its shapes and dimensions, that our inner worlds can be made known through our voices and that the voice can express so much more than the limitations of our own conception of our selves (Pikes, 2005). At first, Wolfsohn believed that Freud's notion of catharsis was the most appropriate framework to explain the therapeutic effects of his teaching. During the second part of this phase, Wolfsohn began to discover the theories of Carl Jung, as he simultaneously grew more confident in his own vocal teaching. Consequently, Wolfsohn began to focus less on facilitating in his students an emotional release through the voice, and more on helping them give vocal expression to mental imagery, including the figures that they reported encountering in their dreams (Gunther, 1990).

7 According to the Jesuit Becker (2001) Jung did a disservice to the Ignatian method since he failed to describe "The Spiritual Exercises" well enough. For a detailed account, see his book *Unlikely Companions: C. G. Jung on the Spiritual Exercises of Ignatius of Loyola*.

Chapter 9

Jungians bridging differences with Desoillians

Jung's failure to acknowledge Robert Desoille and the other guided imagery practitioners, as well as the clear criticism coming from Von Franz, led to the directed waking dream approach to be looked at with suspicion by some prominent classic Jungians and not considered on par with active imagination, as advocated by Jung. This was a missed opportunity for both sides to learn and influence each other's work on the imaginal. However, this was not the case for all Jungians especially those in France and Italy, and those in Uruguay.

One example comes from the late French Jungian analyst, Elie Humbert. He went as far as to question the Jungian dogma that emphasised the importance of staying with the image and not letting it develop freely "but forcing it to keep itself in the form of concrete reality?" (Humbert, 1980, p. 137). Prof. Renos Papadoupulos remembers the heated exchange between Von Franz and Elie Humbert on whether to guide or not to guide imagery in analysis, in the International Congress of Analytical Psychology that took in Rome in 1977 (personal communication).

In France, some Jungians, like Dr. Elie Humbert, Dr. Pierre Solie, Dr. Arthur Arthus[1] and Dr. Jean Pierre Schnetzler, did collaborate with one of Desoille's disciples, such as Dr. Andre Virel who founded an organisation named *Société Internationale* des *Techniques d'Imagerie Mentale* (S.I.T.I.M.), and in 1968 he developed his own directed waking dream method by the name of *Oneirotherapie d'integration* (Virel & Fretigny, 1968). Dr. Jean Pierre Schnetzler had been analysed by Desoille and had trained in this method prior to his training as a Jungian analyst (personal communication on April 16, 2012 from his daughter Elizabeth Schnetzler, a Jungian analyst in Grenoble). All of them published articles in the special edition on mental imagery of the Swiss journal *Action et Pensée* of the Charles Baudouin Institute in 1968. The Jungian Gilberte Aigrisse featured several articles on analytical psychology in several editions of *Action et Penése* in the 50s, 60s, 70s, 80s and 90s. She also wrote a review of Dr. Virel's book "*Histoire de Notre Image*/History of Our Image" in 1967 in the *Journal of Analytical Psychology*.

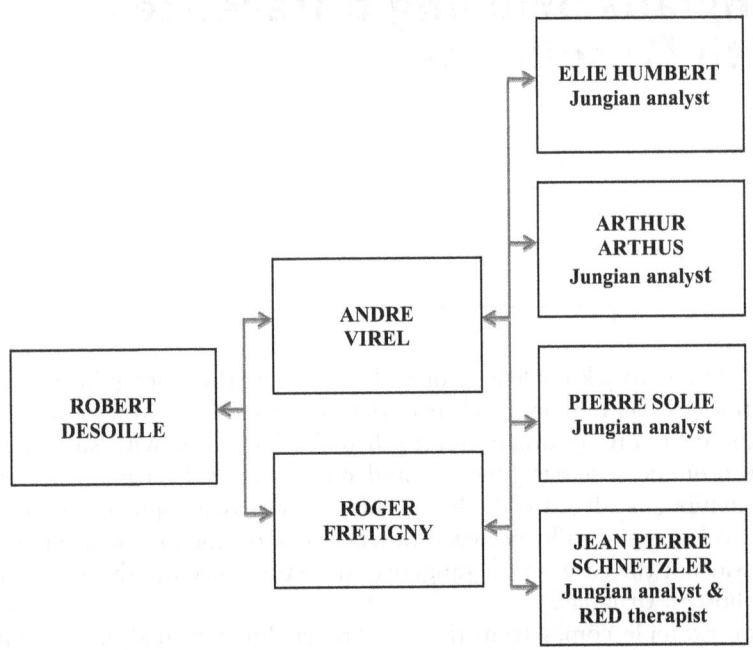

Figure 9.1 French Jungians that collaborated with Desoillians.

Pierre Solie wrote an article titled *"Psychologie analytique et imagerie mental/*Analytical psychology and mental imagery" in 1971 in the third edition of the international journal *Psychotherapies: Revue de l'Arbre Vert*, edited by Dr. Andre Virel, while Dr. Elie Humbert and Dr. Arthur Arthus published *"L'imagination active/*Active imagination" and *"Le fantastique onirique/*Oneiric fantasy" in the fourth and final edition of the same journal in November–December 1971. Dr. Humbert and Dr. Arthus also feature amongst the teaching faculty of the *"Institut d'Enseignement des Methodes Psychotherapiques/*Teaching Institute of Psychotherapeutic Methods" in Paris (founded in 1968), where they taught analytical psychology in this integrative psychotherapy institute with an emphasis on guided imaginative psychotherapy (*Psychotherapies: Revue de l'Arbre Vert, No. 1 & 4, 1971*). They were also involved in the international conferences organised by S.I.T.I.M. Elie Humbert even collaborated in the publication of a dictionary of psychology/psychotherapy by Andre Virel in 1977 entitled *"Dictionnaire de Psychologie: Vocabulaire des Psychothérapie/*Dictionary of Psychology: Vocabulary of Psychotherapy" (personal communication on January 7, 2013).[2] Elie Humbert, Von Franz, Jolande Jacobi, Gilbert Durand and Desoille's friend, Andre Virel, collaborated on a radio programme aired on

August 24, 1970 titled: "*Carl Gustav Jung ou la totalite de l'homme future: Symbole dus soi et individuation*/Carl Gustav Jung or the totality of the man of the future: Symbol of Self and individuation" (personal communication on March 27, 2014).[3] The above-mentioned Jungians acknowledged that in moments of impasse in analysis, the directed waking dream is very effective in helping the patient unblock him- or herself. These words prove what Desoille had previously emphasised *vis-à-vis* the Jungians. Jungians might feel compelled to interfere in the active imagination process as Robert Desoille (1966) said in a lecture at the University of Sorbonne: "Jungian analysts ... have no methods for intentionally evoking [images] so that they can be studied in vivo and used therapeutically" (Desoille, 1966, p. 25).

Unfortunately, the articles by the French Jungians in *Action et Pensée* and the international journal *Psychotherapies: Revue de l'Arbre Vert* were never translated into English after their respective deaths, and French Jungians moved their interest to American and British psychoanalytic theories. Furthermore, before the founding of the French Jungian Society, the *Société Française de Psychologie Analytique* (S.F.P.A.) in 1969, it was frequent that analysts of the Rhône-Alpes area were also members of the Charles Baudouin Institute in Geneva, which also had a centre in Lyon. Dr. Andre Arthus was the key figure in analytical psychology of the Rhône-Alpes area. After his death in 1982, the S.F.P.A. under the direction of President of S.F.P.A. Madame Hélène Wiart-Tebou decided that it was not possible to be a member of both the "Charles Baudouin Institute," which favoured integration of psychoanalytic schools, and the S.F.P.A. (Serina, personal communication; Kirsch, 2000, p. 161). This conceivably marked the end of the mutual formal influence of Desoillians on Jungians. It could very well be that even though the S.F.P.A. has lessened the importance of the "Charles Baudouin institute," the latter's spirit of integration might be the way forward in analytical psychology.

Another example of a Jungian analyst who collaborated with a directed waking dream practitioner is the Swiss Jungian analyst, Jolande Jacobi. She had received a letter dated October 24, 1957 (Hs 1101: 312) from the German psychiatrist, Dr. Hanscarl Leuner, in which he described the lecture he gave at the Jung Club in Zurich and explained his directed waking dream method named "*Katathym Imaginative Psychotherapie*/Guided Affective Imagery." Jacobi liked his presentation. Leuner attaches a detailed manuscript of his method where he asks Jacobi to criticise his work, since it did not always fit a Jungian framework. Leuner's method is very similar to that of Desoille, but Leuner gives ten standard-word stimuli, instead of the six words of Desoille. Leuner was analysed by a Jungian analyst, Dr. Gustav Schmaltz. According to Baeir (2013), the colleague of Dr. Andre Virel, Dr. Roger Fretigny, claimed that both Dr. Hanscarl Leuner and the Jungian Dr. Gustav Heyer were students of the German doctor, Dr. Carl Happich.[4] Leuner[5] was also in correspondence with Jung on April 30, 1959

(Hs 1056: 27045), where he spoke to him about his work on psychosis and his method which he spoke about at the Zurich club and which he developed primarily through the help of Dr. Gustav Schmaltz of Frankfurt.

Furthermore, the renowned late Italian Jungian analyst Dott.ssa Biancha Garufi (1977) wrote an article in the *Journal of Analytical Psychology* on how she worked with a patient in Jungian analysis using elements from the directed day dream of Desoille. In 1978, the late Italian Jungian analyst Dott.ssa Silvana Plateo Zoja wrote her diploma thesis while training at the Jungian Institute of Kusnacht on *Analytical Psychology and Rêve Eveillé Dirigé* which was supervised by Mario Jacobi. Surprisingly, this was the same time when Von Franz was teaching at the same C.G. Jung Institute in Zurich with Mario Jacobi, who was outwardly against directed waking dreams. Dr. Verena Kast of the same Zurich institute also published a book in 1988, *Imagination as Space of Freedom*, on the use of guided imagery in therapy.

One might wonder how Italian analysts got in touch with the directed waking dream. Fortunately, we have some information about Dott.ssa Silvana Plateo Zoja. During the second half of the 60s, the Italian Dr. Maria Robecchi had introduced to Dott.ssa Silvana Plateo Zoja the RED method. Dr. Robecchi was not a psychoanalyst but she used Desoille's method in her practice to induce a relaxing state, a partial hypnosis, to facilitate a healing process and to cope with stress in her medical practice (personal communication).[6] Plateo Zoja also used this technique with her patients, particularly with the ones who did not remember their dreams. One of her patients, a 38-year-old woman, recalled just blurred images with few associations and she spoke in monosyllables. Plateo Zoja decided to attempt a guided daydream and the result after a few REDs was: "[...] she even began to have former dreams [...] her improvement quickened from then on. The RED released the blocked situation" (Plateo-Zoja, 1978, p. 61). In the case of Dott.ssa Biancha Garufi, I have not yet discovered where she had learnt the directed waking dream method.

On the American continent, the late Dr. Mario Berta, a psychiatrist and psychotherapist from Uruguay, had also been analysed by Desoille in Paris in the late 1950s, he helped to introduce the directed waking dream to Uruguay and developed a therapeutic imaginative methodology named "*psicoactivation*/psychoactivation" (Berta, 2001) as well as a projective test called "*L'epreuve d'anticipation*/Anticipation test" (1999). Dr. Berta (1962) also pioneered his research in the 1960s on altered states of consciousness through L.S.D. and used it to induce waking dreams which he named "*Reve eveille lisergico dirigado*/Lysergic directed waking dream." Dr. Berta saw the common imaginative factor in both Jung and Desoille's method and with Dr. Anastasia he summarised the imaginative therapies on the international level (Berta and Anastasia, 2002). In fact, he had met von Franz at the C.G. Jung Institute in Zurich, and practised active imagination besides the directed waking dream with his patients (personal communication from Dr. H. Anastasia, a student of Dr. Berta, on May 1, 2012). One of Berta's close colleagues, Dr. Mario Saiz, was the first president of the C.G. Jung Foundation of Uruguay (Kirsch, 2000).

It seems that Jungians, particularly those in France, were more interested in bridging their approach and dialoguing with Desoillians. They did this with one of Desoille's dissident figures, namely Dr. Andre Virel. It seems that Jungians have preferred to build relationships with those who are not afraid of forging their own identities. It is also understandable that French Jungians would befriend the waking dream methodologies since they knew French.

On a theoretical level, Desoille was influenced and did influence many psychotherapists and psychoanalysts. His integrative spirit can be seen through his activity in the early 50s as a vice president of the "*Société de Recherche de Langue Francaise en Psychotherapie*/French Research Society in Psychotherapy" (Delpech, 1967, p. 10), an umbrella organisation that gathered different schools of thought (including the *Groupe du Rêve-Eveillé-Dirigé en Psychotherapie*) and published a *Bulletin de la S.R.P.L.F.* with a special edition in March 1966, written by Desoille's disciples as a homage after his death during that same year. This organisation formed part of the "International Federation for Medical Psychotherapy,"[7] which since 1991 is the "International Federation for Psychotherapy." Fortunately, Desoille's series of three lectures given at the Sorbonne in January 1965 were translated into English by the American Dr. Frank Haronian and compiled into a booklet titled *Directed Daydream*. As a result, his work finally became slightly more accessible to the English-speaking world, though he did not live long enough to make his work more known at an international level. He died a year later.

The relationship of post-Desoillians to Jung

After Desoille died, his disciples formed an international group of "waking dream" of Desoille (G.I.R.E.D.D. – Groupe International du Rêve-Eveillé-Dirigé de Desoille) in Paris in 1966. After some time, the group's name was changed to G.I.R.E.D. removing the word *dirigé*, i.e., the directivity component, while emphasising spatial movement. However, the group was further divided between those who were in favour of a straightforward entry into psychoanalysis, those who viewed themselves as psychoanalysts but were still true to the original method of Desoille as a way to access the unconscious and the "Desoillians" who believed more in the power of the waking dream itself and who later preferred to identify with Transpersonal and Humanistic schools of thought (Malan, 1975).

The pro-psychoanalytic followers, with respect towards their Desoilian origins, formed G.I.R.E.P. in 1987 (Malan, 1975; Roubineau, 1987).

G.I.R.E.P. has been meeting at *"Le Forum104, espace de rencontre culturel et interspirituel*/Forum 104, a space of cultural and inter-spiritual encounter," at 104, Rue Vaugirard, co-incidentally where the *Club du Gros Caillou,* now known as *"Groupe d'Études C. G. Jung de Paris*/Parisian Study Group on C.G. Jung,"[8] meets as well. G.I.R.E.P. gave their work a post-Freudian approach and remained the main leading group in France. Unfortunately, besides the notion of archetypes, very few Jungian and post-Jungian ideas have been integrated in RED by G.I.R.E.P. with the exception of Descamps[9] (1985, 2004). Jung was and remains a controversial figure in France and has never managed to win a wide popularity there (Thibaudieur, 2011).

Notes

1 Dr. Arthus seemed to have changed his radical view against the directed aspect of the waking dream which he wrote about in the late 1950s and later chose to collaborate with Andre Virel.
2 E-mail sent to me on January 7, 2013 from Jungian analyst Viviane Thibaudieur who spoke with Humbert's wife, Myrtha Humbert, on my behalf.
3 E-mail sent to me by Dr. Vincent Chalmeton, currently responsible for the P.R. of the C.G. Jung Club in Paris, told me what he found. The programme was the third series on C.G. Jung presented by B. Latour and the introduction of the radio programme can be found on the website of INA radio station: www.ina.fr/audio/PHD99213327.
4 Carl Happich mentioned that he was in discussion with Heyer in a letter he sent to Jung on May 14, 1934 (Ref no: HS 1056:2781).
5 Leuner seems to have also influenced the work of the late American music therapist, Helen Bonny (1978), who developed a guided imagery approach through music in the 60s. She called her music therapy approach "Guided Imagery and Music" (G.I.M.). She adapted Leuner's ten verbal stimuli to pieces of music. Her work was also influenced by Freud, Jung, Maslow, Assagioli and Desoille.
6 E-mail sent to me by Dott.ssa Sara Zoja, daughter of Dott.ssa Silvana Plateo Zoja, on March 10, 2014.
7 This was previously known as the "International General Medical Society for Psychotherapy." In 1928, Jung became a member of this Society. He was elected vice president in 1930 and was asked to take up its presidency in 1933, which he did in 1934 (Gallard, 1994). It was re-established as the "International Federation for Medical Psychotherapy" in 1958 with Medard Boss as its president.
8 It is commonly known as "The Paris Jungian club."
9 He was a didactic member of G.I.R.E.P. and also a founder of the French Transpersonal Association. He died in December 2018.

Part III

Comparing RED and active imagination

Chapter 10

The concept of interiority and its development in Western Europe

The notion of interiority has a long history in the Western world (Foucault, 1986; Taylor, 1989; Cary, 2000). Transformation is often experienced and described as a process of turning inwards. The idea of interiority is a precursor of the concept of the inner self-experience, which was eventually absorbed into psychology. Diaries of early Greek philosophers, along with autobiographies and biographies of religious people, which focus on inner life, are in fact the forerunners of modern psychological introspection and analysis. The particular interior dimension of both Jung's and Desoille's psychological discourse helps to shape and distinguish their own waking dream methods. Moreover, their emphasis offers an essential vantage point for deliberating over a remaking of their own lives. Both offer a theoretical paradigm, suggesting that inward movement from world to self is to be understood merely not as a regressive retreat into oneself, but as a movement that leads into deeper levels of relatedness to the world and other people. It is an inward movement of awareness that reaches into and through one's own core. This inward movement of awareness eventually leads towards an outward release of energy from that core. Both Jung and Desoille physically exteriorised psychic space into a public arena through their writings about their imaginative methods. In fact, both Jung's autobiographical account of his own active imagination in *The Red Book* and Desoille's biographical accounts of his patient's *rêve éveillé*'s resonate well with other classic personal accounts in devotional literature such as St. Augustine's *Confessions* and St. Teresa of Ávila's *The Interior Castle* amongst others, which were the means of physically unfolding their private inscapes into a public arena.

In fact, in both methods there is a dialectical movement between interior and exterior, secrecy and revelation, image and word, aloneness and presence. However, at times, interiority has been idealised in the case of Jung's active imagination and literalised in the case of Desoille to the extent that it has limited the development of both techniques from further developing and updating with the times. Current psychological language is characterised by new contemporary discourse which has superceded the interior-exterior divide and which reflects changes in social, political, technological and economic issues. Hence, we would expect that the development of the waking dream methods would also centre on a new "interior" trope.

To begin with, I would like to explain the common understanding that exists when it comes to the meaning of the word "interior." It usually refers to an inner space or dimension, a place which contains the inner self, the true being of the person. The concept of a psychological interior is meant to refer to the idea that a person has within themselves a space, into which one may subjectively turn to, and not a feature that can be examined from without or in any physical manner. The word "interior" connotes a localised centre of awareness bounded by the physical body and which is in turn surrounded by an unbounded field of extensional space. The notion of interiority is nowadays frequently associated with the discipline of psychology. However, it is also present in other disciplines such as philosophy[1] and spirituality[2] but maybe not to the extent of psychology. Jesus in the New Testament described an ethic of self-improvement which goes as far back to the ancient Greeks. The Gospel says: "It is from within, from the human heart, that evil intentions come" (Matt 7, 18).

Historical and philosophical studies in relation to the "interior" include those of Foucault (1986), Taylor (1989) and Cary (2000). Michel Foucault (1989) traces the development of modern identity to Augustine (354–430 AD), describing him as the innovator of our modern sense of "inwardness" and the "interior," now embedded in modern reflexive language. Cary (2000) highlights the contribution of Plotinus (232–304 CE) on interiority. The "interior" that Plotinus describes is a medium between soul and God, and is quite different from our modern psychological "interior." The major insight of Taylor's (1989) *Sources of the Self* is that modern subjectivity has its roots in ideas of human good. Taylor shows that the modern turn inward is not disastrous but is in fact the result of our long efforts to define and reach the good.

In Western culture, there is a long tradition about the ancient notion of the "cultivation of the self," a lifelong process of acquiring self-knowledge (Foucault, 1989). For the Stoics, the care of the self became an internalised procedure, where one internally reflects to get a sense of truth. The Stoics developed the notions of self-care and self-discovery into a discipline of *askesis* (Foucault, 1986, p. 51). St. Augustine's *Confessions* is a personal account of his own inner conversion to Christianity and can be considered as the first Western autobiography ever written, which became an influential model for Christian writers throughout the following 1000 years of the Middle Ages. Furthermore, the Christian monastic ascetic tradition of the Early Church, which started in Eastern Europe before moving to the West, focused on meditation on the Holy Scriptures so as to reach perfection. In the High Middle Ages (1000–1300 CE), mystics such as Hildegard of Bingen, Bernard of Clairvaux and Bonaventure, and later the Beguine mystics and the mystics of the Rhineland such as Meister Eckhart, Johann Tauler and Henry Suso in the Late Middle Ages (1300–1500 CE) contributed to a personal experience of faith in God through contemplative prayer which led to many visions of union with God. Their inner fervour and practice of finding the heart spread from the monk, the troubadour, and the saint, to the common person. The lay citizens were encouraged to look into their own hearts for their source of spirituality. All of this suggested a movement towards the humanistic, that is, a looking within oneself, rather than to an outside authority, for the source of knowing.

In the seventeenth century, the "inner man" metamorphosed into the "invisible," and the "interior" described by Augustine in his *Confessions*, was located at the "bottom" of one's "heart." Indeed, the bottom (*le fond*) and the deep (*le profond*) were exchanged during translation with Augustine's original terms of *fundus* (*a fundo cordis mei*/bottom of my heart), *intimo cordis* (inmost heart) as well as *intus* (inside). This confusion of terms took place after the series of French translations[3] and editions of the original *Confessions* of St. Augustine such as the translations of Artaud d'Andilly (1649), Philippe Goibaud du Bois (1686) and Simon-Michel Treuve (1703). The spiritual landscape of the seventeenth century shifted from scholastic authority to more experiential spirituality from the mind to the heart. Pascal's dictum *"le coeur a ses raisons que la raison ne connait point*/the heart has reasons which reason knows not" is perhaps the best-known expression of what at the time of the *Pensees*[4] was becoming a devotional commonplace (Papasogli, 1991). Moreover, the idea of depth and interiority connoted not only the rhetoric of sin but also the positive language of affective mysticism which promised plenitude with every turn. The *Confessions* then emerged in the seventeenth century as a book with two interrelated concepts of interiority, namely the interior as dark centre of the secretive subject but also the interior as the burning, experiential heart visited by mystics. Mysticism was no longer for the few who had been schooled in the theology of Pseudo-Dionysius or Tauler, but became an experience for those without knowledge of Christianity's great mystical works. The popularizing of mysticism can be observed in the mutations of two keywords in seventeenth-century spirituality, words that gradually lost their theological importance even as they were provoking more enthusiasm in devotional literature. These words were interior *"interieur*/interior" and *"coeur*/heart." Devotional literature moved away from the Augustinian distinction between exterior man, i.e., the part of man also shared by animals such as perception, and interior man referring to faculties which animals do not have such as reason. Instead, interior came to designate a vague psychological space to which logic, reason and even language were foreign, indeed exterior (Paige, 2001).

The Church's position started to include the role of human emotion in gaining an understanding of God. In the past, the Church had emphasised intellect as a means of gaining religious truth, and rays of light emanating from the heart had symbolised revelation through reason. Following St. Teresa of Avila's vision, the heart pierced by an arrow, which symbolised revelation through emotion, came into greater prominence. At this point, the interior disappeared from theological discourse, and became instead an essential part of devotional literature, literature intended for consumption by a wider audience rather than the clerical male readership of theology. The heart comes to symbolise the spontaneity of our being, not subject to logical, rational and non-discursive contemplation. This was also seen in Protestantism which is commonly viewed as stressing inner devotion over external ritual. The late seventeenth-century reform movement known as Pietism[5] represented an intensification of Lutheran inwardness that had long-lasting cultural effects, especially in Northern Germany. Pietism altered the religious and the linguistic landscape by transmitting its soul-searching vocabulary to the eighteenth century's culture of sensibility.

In literature, literary figures became increasingly enamoured with their innermost depths. Like Goethe's troubled protagonist Werther,[6] readers thrived on the relentless self-examination such characters undertook. By the turn of the century, metaphors of depth and inwardness saturated the prose of authors such as Novalis, Wackenroder, Tieck and Jean Paul (Draaisma, 2000; Watkins, 2011). The breadth of meanings that those metaphors evoked in the 1800s rivalled those of religious discourse circa 1675. Taking Pietism's emphasis on subjective experience to its limit, Romantic thinkers invested the self with qualities usually reserved for the divine – unknowability, unscrutability, even infinity. Watkins writes: "By merging the divine and human they transformed the inner realm from a private site of prayer and reflection into an unfathomable abyss" (Watkins, 2011, p. 29). While Pietists believed that the inward journey ultimately reached the divine, their romantic counterparts tended to stray further and further into the fathomless depths of subjective interiority.

All the above philosophical, theological and literary traditions of interiority in the Western world were steeped in the works of both Jung and Desoille and can be identified if one looks closely at the metaphors chosen to describe the internal landscapes. A close look at Jung's *The Red Book* reveals the frequent citations of St. Paul, St. Augustine, Meister Eckhart, Thomas a Kempis, Jacob Boehme, Swedenborg, Joseph von Görres and Jeanne Guyon amongst others, while Desoille makes reference to St. Augustine, St. Denis the Areopagite, Blaise Pascal, St. Theresa of Avila and St John of the Cross, and Therese Neuman in his 1938 book. Desoille also references the work of the psychoanalyst John Leuba (1925) *"Psychologie du Mysticisme Religieux*/Psychology of Religious Mysticism," the book of the Jesuit Joseph Marechal (1924) *"Etudes sur la Psycholgie des Mystiques*/Studies on the Psychology of Mystics," *"De l'Angoise à l'Ecstase*/From Angst to ecstasy" of Pierre Janet (1927) and the work of William James (1906) *"Les Variétés de l'Expérience Religieuse*/The Varieties of Religious Experience," who were open to mystical experiences. Desoille's position, despite his strong scientific attitude, does not pathologise mystic experiences and values their creative and transformational aspects. Desoille also writes the preface of the book of the philosopher Genevieve Lanfranchi "*De la vie interieure à la vie de relation*/From the interior life to the relational life," where he argues that psychology can see mystic states in a positive healthy way (Desoille, 1966). Desoille and Jung's respective ideas about the transpersonal seem to have been on the same lines.

Notes

1 Amongst philosophers for example, phenomenologists such as Husserl, Heidegger and Sartre look for philosophical truth in the human interiority just as Descartes did before them, although most of them do not accept Cartesian rationalism (Pivcevic, 1970).

2 A spirituality of interiority can be found in the Catholic *Devotio moderna* of Thomas a Kempis, the "Spiritual Exercises" of St. Ignatius of Loyola and the devotional practices of apostolic religious orders. In modern times, the Catholic retreat house became the central Catholic place of spirituality of interiority (Griffin, Beardslee and Holland, 1989).

3 For a detailed account of the changes in translations of St. Augustine's *Confessions*, see Nicholas D. Paige's (2001) book *Being Interior: Autobiography and Contradiction of Modernity in Seventeenth Century France* and Matthew W. Maguire's (2006) book *The Conversion of Imagination: From Pascal through Rousseau to Tocqueville*.

4 The *Pensées* which means "thoughts" is a collection of fragments on theology and philosophy written by seventeenth-century French philosopher and mathematician Blaise Pascal. Pascal's religious conversion led him into a life of asceticism and the *Pensées* was in many ways his life's work (Copleston, 1958).

5 Pietism refers to an influential religious reform movement that began amongst German Lutherans in the seventeenth century. It emphasised personal faith against the main Lutheran church's perceived stress on doctrine and theology over Christian living. Pietism quickly spread and later became concerned with social and educational matters. As a phenomenon of personal religious renewal, its indirect influence has persisted in Germany and other parts of Europe into the twenty-first century. Two important scholarly books on the subject are F. Ernest Stoeffler's 1965 book *The Rise of Evangelical Pietism* and Douglas H. Shantz's 2013 work entitled *An Introduction to German Pietism: Protestant Renewal at the Dawn of Modern Europe*.

6 Werther is a fictional character in Johann Wolfgang von Goethe's epistolary, loosely autobiographical novel *The Sorrows of Young Werther*, first published in 1774.

Chapter 11

On spatial metaphors of interiority

While sharing a common goal, that of a return to oneself, the path to wholeness led Jung and Desoille down separate roads, which converge at times through their linguistic symbolism and spatial metaphors. Both of them use specific internal spatial language and tropes when engaging in their waking dream techniques. In this section, I will be focusing on the idea of spatial metaphors used in describing interiority to compare the Jungian technique with Desoille's method. In choosing spatiality as a comparative tool, I am following recent scholarship in several disciplines which have become increasingly spatial in their orientation. These include such fields as literary and cultural studies, sociology, political science, sociology, anthropology, history and religion (Nora, 1984; Soja, 1989, 1996; Lefebvre, 1991; Massey, 1994, 1995, 2005; Bourdieu, 2000; Bordwell and Thompson, 2008). The American Professor of Geography Denis Cosgrove refers to this shift as a "spatial turn" (Cosgrove, 1999, p. 7) while the French philosopher Michel Foucault (1986), in a lecture given in 1967, argues how the great obsession of the nineteenth century with history and its temporal stages of development have given way to "the epoch of space."

Jung and Desoille share a common goal that of a return to oneself, yet the path to wholeness led them down separate roads which, it may be argued, converge at times through their linguistic symbolism and spatial metaphors. The language and metaphors of inwardness are built into our psychological and epistemological language so intimately that we have literally embodied them. According to Lakoff and Johnson (1980), conceptual understanding is, in fact, structured by metaphors. Lakoff and Johnson also argue that metaphorical concepts structure how we perceive the world and, as such, create reality.

In fact, in both methods there is a dialectical movement between interior and exterior, secrecy and revelation, image and word, aloneness and presence. However, at times, interiority has been idealised in the case of Jung's active imagination and literalised in the case of Desoille to the extent that it has limited the development of both techniques from further developing and updating with the times. Current psychological language is characterised by new contemporary discourse which has superceded the interior-exterior divide and which reflects changes in social, political, technological and economic issues. Hence, we would expect that the development of the waking dream methods would also centre on a new "interior" trope.

Spatial metaphors on interiority in Jung's and Desoille's accounts of waking dreams

Aristotle tied down the notion of place in his *Physics* to that of a merely bounded space when he argues that place is the inner limit of a containing body. Space was robbed of substantive meaningfulness to become an ordered, uniform system of abstract linear co-ordinates. This was further reinforced by Newton and Galileo's claims of an infinite and infinitely open space. In their methods, space offered a means for measuring time; therefore, space was subordinate to time, and the importance of place largely forgotten. The French philosopher Gaston Bachelard (1964), in his *Poetics of Space*, has produced an experiential account of our lived spaces. Bachelard renewed the mytho-poetic idea of inner place, when he posited that the invisible is revealed in the interiority of the human soul and, as such, it is intrinsically a place. Such an idea of psychological space makes up for the impoverished one of Euclidean and Newtonian space. Likewise, both Jung and Desoille claimed that creative action of the poetic imagination provides an abode of intimate immensity that mirrors the external immensity of the cosmos, and provides a space capable of a marvellous transformation. However, it was Hillman who clearly deconstructed the notions of an interior space and place where somehow both Jung and Desoille are caught in. For Hillman, the sense of "in-ness" refers neither to location nor to physical containment: "[...] but an imaginal metaphor for the soul's non-visible and non-literal inherence, the imaginal psychic quality within all events" (Hillman, 1975, p. 173).

However, in this chapter I will be keeping to Jung's and Desoille's "traditional topology" of inner space and place and will choose to focus more on their choice of tropes and on an inner spatio-analysis of the workings of their methods.

Altitudo: on spatial vertical dialectics

Jung and Desoille's methods encourage the patient to go inside and to imagine the inside as it were an outside and to experience it. For both of them, the interior place is not just the closed small world of one's intimacies. It can also be an infinite challenging universe which man can chart. In fact, the theme of *"homo viator/*man on the way"[1] is an archetypal one and features considerably in classic authors such as Plotinus, Homer, Virgil, Valmiki and Dante (Papasogli, 1991; De Waal, 1993). Jung describes wandering as "a symbol for longing, of the restless urge which never finds its object, of nostalgia for the lost mother" (Jung, 1912/1967, p. 205 [CW5, para. 299]). However, the preferred road maps for the peregrination are not the same. Several times, the adventures do not unfold horizontally but are played vertically. The vertical axis, in Latin *altitudo*, extends between ultimate heights and ultimate depths and incorporates both. Gaping altitude or culminating depth, the extreme acuminal and the extreme abyssal meet and coincide.

In our Western literary tradition, there has been emphasis on "anabasis," i.e., ascents. In the alchemical tradition, the Sky and the Earth are the vertical alchemical couple and *axis mundi* corresponding to the horizontal Brother-Sister couple. The accent can be put on one or the other. Since Plato's *Phaedrus* where he describes the loss of wings of the soul and its subsequent fall, further echoed in the myths of Icarus and Bellorophon, there remains a yearning and nostalgia for unity with that which is above. In the Platonic tradition, the above *logos* outside the cave is the sole truth and below is the murky shadow. Bachelard's book *L'Air et les Songes* (1943) further idealised the aerial heights and later the fire of the imagination. Man carries in himself an inclination, something like a tropism towards his eternal origin.

The above concepts have been challenged by postmodernism.[2] Derrida speaks about plunging into "the horizontality of a pure surface" (Derrida, 1978, p. 28) and that for deconstructionists everything is surface, appearance, horizontality. Not only do deconstructionists deny absolute transcendence, but even relative height or depth (Jameson, 1991). Such views took the place of modernism's dualistic models of depth and surface, essence and appearance, latent and manifest, authenticity and inauthenticity, signified and signifier (ibid., p. 12). While surface is essential for both Jung and Desoille in order to bring back the images which are met in the depths and heights, the unconscious remains central to both practitioners.

Interior wet suits and interior space suits

Following a Kantian epistemology, Jung holds that one cannot tell what the psyche is but one can only say how it appears to us without concluding that it is how it is in itself. Jung's psychology is based on soul and a being in soul (*esse in anima*). For Jung, all we know about the world is in images, since that is how psyche presents itself directly. Jung chooses to represent the psyche's depths, which he himself has chosen to face. Like a Surrealist *flâneur*, Jung inserts himself into the anonymous figures and landscape of the depths. He thus exemplifies the historical shift from *Gemeinschaft* to *Gesellshaft* by trying his best to feel at home in the crowd of strangers of the unconscious. For Jung, in *The Red Book*: "the inner is as infinite as the world of the outer [...] and is no way poorer than the outer one"

(Jung, 2009, p. 264). Jung moves from the external sensitive faculties to the fine bottom of the heart, from top downwards and from outside towards the interior: "He whose desires turn away from outer things reaches the place of the soul" (ibid., p. 232). From the periphery towards the centre, towards this mysterious depths called "desert," "abyss," "Hell" (from Latin *locus infernos* meaning the place beneath), "bottommost," "immeasurable depths." Jung describes how one's being "pulls you to the bottom like lead" (ibid., p. 266).

Consequently, Jung demolishes and reverses a European tradition which idealises ascents and is resistant to the fall, towards an embracing of descents: "Let fall what wants to fall; if you stop it, it will sweep you away" (Jung, 2009, p. 244). Jung describes how the spirit of the depths approached him and said: "Climb down into your depths, sink" (ibid., p. 240), since he has been too much in the summits. In the 1925 seminar, Jung (1925/1989, p. 63) recounted how the first time he practised active imagination, he had reached a depth of about 1,000 feet and later when he tried it again he went much deeper. Jung subverses the principles which have governed the space of intimacy before him. In order for this to be achieved, Jung had to descend to the very lowest of himself and embrace all that was inferior in himself.

In *The Red Book*, Jung peregrinates through various underground caves as well as horizontal places, such as deserts in which he finds fertile fields, gardens, libraries and lodges. The dryness and light of the desert, which we are introduced to in *The Red Book*, contrasts sharply with the darkness of the sea. Jung uses the metaphor of the sea and the night to describe the inner depths. Jung attributes the term "night sea journey" to Frobenius, to whose extensive study of myths Jung refers in the *Collected Works* (Jung, 1912/1967, p. 210 [*CW5*, para. 308]). The night sea journey or *Nekyia* is a recurring cross-cultural ancient mythical theme which reappears, relatively more recently, again and again in the fairy tales and legends of the dragon-slaying heroes. Moreover, darkness and night time should not always be associated with the shadows of evil, for it provides the opportunity for the most intense contemplation. It can be a time of sorrow, as it was for Job; however, the anguish led to deliverance. Moreover, it was during the night that Christ came into the world, and it is at night that salvation can be attained. These themes of the nocturnal sea appear again and again in the *Collected Works*, from *Symbols of Transformation* (1912/1967) through to *Mysterium Coniunctionis* (1955/1970).

In *The Red Book*, Jung describes man as a "drop in the ocean" who "wander[s] vast distances in blurred currents and [...] [is] swept back into the depths" (Jung, 2009, p. 266). Jung's references to the night sea journey also parallel those of French seventeenth-century moralist and devotional literature for whom the sea trope with its rough seas and forceful winds was a metaphor of man's search and journey towards God. These sea metaphors reflect the vastness of the outer world which also belongs inside. These metaphors are inspired by the geographical discoveries of the new worlds by the European powers (Papasogli, 1991; Gross & Gross, 1993). Furthermore, the image of man lost at sea connotes man's alienation from God. The passions are also associated with rough seas which man has to try to sail through without drowning in them (Papasogli, 1991).

Jung uses the images of the *Nekyia* (the night sea journey) and *Katabasis* (descent into the lower world) almost interchangeably. In the *Visions Seminars* (1930–1934), Jung explains how, in ancient times, people would go to down to the "oracular cave" or to "a hidden spring" since the secret place of initiation was below (Jung, 1998, p. 92). James Hillman, however, made some clear distinctions between *Nekyia* and *Katabasis*:

> The descent of the underworld can be distinguished from the night sea-journey of the hero in many way […] the hero returns from the night sea-journey in better shape for the tasks of life, whereas the nekyia takes the soul into a depth for its own sake so that there is no 'return.'
>
> (Hillman, 1979, p. 88)

In the case of Desoille, the vertical line determines the anthropological structure of the human being. Both Jung and Desoille agree that the structures of above and below were not made up but both believe in their archetypal basis. Jung even says that Dante intuited this when he wrote his opus of the *Divine Comedy*. For Desoille (1938), the heights are almost always connected with good feelings while the depths evoke fear and primitive anxiety. Desoille makes use of the symbol of the descent, but puts greater emphasis on that of the ascent. In Desoille's directed waking dream, Desoille also does encourage the patient to go down. Eventually, the descent to the cave becomes one of his main initial stimuli when Desoille tried to give more structure to his approach. The experience of going down many times becomes a maritime one. The patients face the dark depths of the sea and they undergo several underwater explorations. Desoille encourages his patients to wear wet-suits and to face the dangerous sea monsters which hinder them from exploring further. He even provides his patients with magical solutions of how to overwhelm the menacing figures. In Desoille's case studies, he mentions several times how his patients are afraid of going down and how he has to encourage them to explore the space above by jumping on a rainbow or a ray of light or cloud, which transports them on higher planes where many times they find fields of gold, rich palaces, saintly and angelic figures and dazzling light.

Desoille (1938) gives more descriptions of the heights rather than the depths and after the patient experiences the heights more frequently, the figures encountered usually shift to an experience of being enveloped by light. Desoille's bias towards the heights has been fuelled from the writings on the five writings on the "material imagination" of his close friend, philosopher Gaston Bachelard (1943), who used the Empedocles' doctrine of the four elements as the roots and "*hormone*/hormones" of the psyche. One can appreciate how networking can lead to sharing and influencing of ideas. Bachelard writes about the material, movement, will and intimacy of imagination in his five books on the imagination. He dedicates the fourth chapter of *L'Air et les Songes* to Desoille where he equates imagination with "*mouvement*/movement." Bachelard was heavily influenced by Jung's text *Psychology and Alchemy* and by the French psychoanalytic pioneer Rene Allendy (1889–1942), who was very much interested in alchemy and Jung's work. Bachelard makes a close link between poetry and alchemy. Novalis is more the poet of fire, Edgar Alan Poe of water, Nietzsche of air, while Goethe is the poet of the earth (Chiore, 2004). Jung also seems to be following Goethe in his metaphorical descriptions on the inner depths. In his *Pilgrim's Progress*, Jung says that it consisted of having to go down a "thousand ladders" to reach out to the "little clod of earth that I am" (Jung, 1973, p. 19). In *Memories, Dreams, Reflections* (1963/1995), Jung is quoted by Jaffe as saying that he needed to materialise the images of his waking dreams in stone by building his tower in Bollingen. Here Jung seems to be echoing the lyrical writings of the French philosopher Roger Callois (1970) "*L'Ecriture des Pierres*/The Writing of Stones." Jung's ideas of having to use one's will to face the images so that ultimately one can find some rest are also elaborated in Bachelard's (1948) works, namely "*La Terre et les Reveries de la Volonte: Essai sur l'Imagination des Forces/ Earth and Reveries of Will: An Essay on the Imagination of Strength.*" For Bachelard the will to "hammer" the earth into new forms brings energy to what is seemingly inert. Working wilfully with the hands on matter energises the imagination to create something new and enliven that substance.

If we use the interpretation given by the post-Jungian James Hillman (1979) on the difference between soul and spirit, we can maybe position both waking dream approaches better. Hillman distinguishes between soul and spirit since soul is the lost dimension in the tripartite structure of human nature, namely spirit, soul and body. So while peaks are associated with the search for spirit or the drive of the spirit in search of itself, vales are connected to depressive moods. Hillman emphasises the fact not to try to liberate the soul from the vale so as to reach transcendence and neither to reduce the spirit to a complex. To the contrary, one must aim for a marriage, a *coniunctio* between the high-driving spirit and the soul, between Eros and Psyche. Hillman argues how the soul can contain, nourish, and elaborate and deepen in fantasy the *puer* impulse, while the soul's reflections need to be seen through in terms of higher and deeper perspectives. In this context, Desoille's directed waking dream emphasises more the spiritual element. Desoille's emphasis on light imagery connotes the last stages of the *via mystica*, namely the *via illuminativa* and the *via contemplativa*, where there is union with God. Furthermore, some of his initial stimuli, such as the road, the mountain, the stairway and the ladder, are all metaphors which mystics mention in their progress of union with the Divine being. Furthermore, the absorption of Desoille's directed waking dream in the 1970s into psychosynthesis, which gives more emphasis to higher consciousness, is more proof of Desoille's spiritual bias.

Jung chooses to keep both the two poles. In *The Red Book*, Jung's (2009) ka-soul came from below, out of the earth, slightly demonic, while the almost God-like spirit Philemon appeared from above in the sky, as if both soul and spirit were inspired by the image of a bird. Moreover, *The Red Book* has several references to the ascetic spiritual practices of the Desert fathers or anchorites although it gives considerable importance to earthly horizontal journey and peregrinations to the bowels of the earth. For Jung in individuation, one aims for the attainment of full knowledge of the heights and depths of one's character.

Confronting the depths directly or facing them gradually?

Jung and Desoille both agree to face one's inferior parts; however, they differ in the approach used. For Jung, the psyche's odyssey to reconquer its unity is very tortuous and the right way to wholeness is a *longissima via* a painful experience of the union of opposites. It is a *discensus ad inferos*. At one point in *The Red Book* in the *Liber Primus*, Jung describes how "Elijah climbs before me into the heights to a very high summit, I follow him" (Jung, 2009, p. 251). Jung explains this move as his resistance to go down. His stronger tendency was to go up since: "on the heights, [...] you are your best, and you become aware only of your best, [...] [and] on the heights, imagination is at its strongest" (ibid., p. 266). Jung further adds: "Your values want to draw you away from what you presently are, to get you ahead and beyond yourself" (ibid.).

So for Jung one cannot arrive to the heights prematurely since it would be an escape into becoming before one fully immerses into his depth of being which is the "bath of rebirth" (ibid., p. 266). However, one can move from experiencing the depths (being) to soaring to the heights (becoming), since both are possible. He writes: "your way leads you from mountain to valley and from valley to mountain" (ibid., p. 266).

Desoille finds very little difficulty in stopping the descents and offers the patient shelter in the waking dream by encouraging him or her to ascend to a higher place. While in Jung's *Red Book*, we can almost hear him shiver with fear of looking inwards, nonetheless, he soldiers on alone. In *Memories, Dreams, Reflections* and in Shamdasani's (1996) introduction to *The Psychology of Kundalini Yoga*, Jung does describe how, when faced with terrifying moments, he would stop to do some actual breathing exercises before returning again to the depths. In fact, in *The Red Book*, he faces the Red One as well as the terrifying Izdubar on his own. Even though Jung recommends active imagination after going through a process of analysis, and therefore after having strengthened one's ego, he still warns against the dangers of being overwhelmed by the unconscious. The unsuccessful descent to Hades by Pirithous is a case in point. Moreover, the allegory of the Sorcerer's Apprentice contains a warning of how easy it is to make the waters gush out, but how difficult it then is to control them and command them back. Desoille is very aware of this and he goes about it in a very supportive manner. Jung's waking dreams are very much non-directive while Desoille takes a more directive approach. Moreover, the presence of the therapist seems to provide holding for the patient in moments of distress and the voicing of the oneirodrama to the therapist serves as an anchor when charting rough seas.

Waiting for or instilling movement of psychic energy

Jung argues that the energies of the psyche seek to move forwards, a movement from within outwards. The psyche projects this process foreword by means of images which can provide possibilities of what may be fulfilled in the outer life. However, at times when this movement is blocked, instead of the psychic energy moving forwards and outwards, it moves backwards and downwards. The energies of the psyche not only go downwards into the depths, but also go backwards into the past. In his essay *On Psychic Energy*, Jung describes the descent of the hero on his underworld journey as the "symbolical exponent of the movement of libido" (Jung, 1948/1960, p. 36 [CW8, para. 68]). The psyche draws on repressed material from the past and unused potential to resolve the current impasse. So the reason that the energies of the psyche move into the past is not because they are caught there by repression. It is a question of finding in the individual's past experiences and archetypal material in the depths of the psyche, ideas with which to encounter the current problem so as to move into the future.

In the *Visions Seminars* (1930–1934), Jung explains how the mobilisation of psychic energy is heralded by images which show "independent, autonomous movement" (Jung, 1998, p. 107). He also adds that some of his patients pictured this surge of autonomous psychic energy "by a green shoot, or a plant which unfolds perhaps two leaves" (ibid., p. 111). He also makes reference to astrological symbols such as Aries and Taurus, whose ram and bull are symbols of fertility and growth (ibid., p. 110).

Desoille also speaks of psychic energy clearly borrowing terminology from Pierre Janet, who also had influenced Jung significantly. Desoille speaks of the elimination of the dissociation between the consciousness and the lower unconscious, which has been produced by repression and how the super-ego limits the development of sublime potential of the patient's Self. Desoille's method clearly demonstrates the loss of libido, especially when patients cannot make the ascents. Nonetheless, he provides them with a catalyst so that they can transform and sublimate their negative emotions and inner states to more positive ones.

Sublimation: Jungian and Desoillian perspectives

In *The Tavistock Lectures*, Jung (1935/1976) describes how "The descent into the depths will bring healing" (Jung, 1935/1976, p. 123 [CW18, para. 270]). Healing is compared to an alchemical process of *sublimatio*: "that it is recognized and made an object of conscious discrimination" (Jung, 1955/1970, p. 204 [CW14, para. 262]).

Jung refers to the union of spirit and soul, reason and feeling, intellect and eros as the *unio mentalis* (ibid., p. 497). In order to reach an *unio mentalis*, one has to reach a reconciliation of opposites. These opposites have to be separated if they are to be reunited at a higher level. The aim of this separation is to free the mind from the influence of the bodily appetites. Man has to face his or her shadow.[3] This leads at first to a dissociation of the personality through a process of introversion and introspection. Psychologically, *sublimatio* is associated with dissociation. Edinger describes the ability of the psyche to dissociate as "both the source of ego-consciousness and the cause of mental illness" (Edinger, 1985, p. 126). Therefore, dissociation can be considered pathological when it gets out of control. However, dissociation can also refer to the sense of detachment from an engulfment in one's personal issues and the possibility to view them objectively. At times, this is healthy and not pathological. According to Edinger (1985), one can set aside one's unconscious identification with complexes and become aware of the far more expansive underlying Self.

In alchemical imagery, sublimation was often depicted as a bird escaping from a person who was undergoing an ordeal. There are a few more symbols that appear in alchemical literature as well as in dreams associated with sublimation. Such symbols include the tower and the mountain-top. Rising to heaven is another symbol for *sublimation*.[4] Typically, one experiences *sublimatio* and then returns to earth, a *coagulatio* process, to live out and integrate what has been learned from the archetypes. The Emerald Tablet also directs us to ascend from earth to heaven, and again return to earth, and unite together the powers of higher things and lower things.

This leads to the reuniting of the *unio mentalis* with the body, from where the complete conjunction be attained, i.e., the union with the *unus mundus*. The reuniting of the spiritual position with the body, which is considered the second stage of conjunction, obviously means that the insights gained should be made real, as one should do in the final stage of active imagination.

However, Desoille sees his RED method as a means of sublimating negative emotions into positive ones and releasing the potential of every patient. In his essay, *The Energies of Men*, William James (1907) draws attention to a number of energy potentialities existing in man, waiting to be discovered,

activated and used. Desoille's method offers a way of activating these energies and for the ego to unite with the higher Self, which he calls a repression
of the sublime. For Desoille, facing the descents is one way of weakening the
negative injunctions of the super-ego which takes the shape of several negative images which block the way of the patient, preventing ascendance. Desoille encourages the patient to face these negative figures so as to transform
them into more benign figures. Desoille directs the patients upwards towards
an ascent from the Latin *ad scandare*, step by step. The ascent, directed by
the analyst, becomes a reward for an *ascesis* (discipline), not in the sense of
ascetism but in the Greek psychagogic sense of psycho-spiritual development.

Desoille is more directive in stimulating movement in the imagination since he believes that movement will result in a change of the heavy
emotional states, a release of a creative force in the patient and an ability to reach ascents more easily. This experience is very similar to Jung's
transcendent function[5] which leads to a complete transformation of the
person. Incidentally, Jung's friend Herman Keyserling (1938) speaks of a
dimension of "intensity," associating the symbolism of intensification with
that of proceeding along a different dimension which he terms "vertical."
In using this term, he is referring to a "verticality" that rises from the world
of becoming, towards the world of being and transcendence. The instant
in front of a menacing figure or aura of light becomes a sudden source of
consciousness which calls for an acute act of attention. Such moments or
augunblick of transformation awaken us to a sur-reality beyond ordinary
notions of the real. In the "aha" moment, the temporal sense of a "before"
and an "after" dissolves to reveal a new moment of personal insight. It frees
us from the ineluctable flow of *durée*.

However, while in Jung's *Red book* we can see the considerable number
of days that would pass before Jung engages in a waking dream (as seen
from the gaps in the entry dates of Jung's active imagination dialogues in
the *Red Book*) to ultimately reach some form of integration, in Desoille
there is a quicker process in achieving change. In Desoille's directed waking dream method, less patience seems to be needed in contrast to Jung's
arduous and timely process in active imagination. Moreover, in Jung's case,
transformation is more a question of grace rather than will. So if the spatial
imagery is not completely different, the time factor seems to provide a main
difference in the two waking dream methods. While Jung's active imagination takes place after a period of analysis and can be an on-going practice,
Desoille underlines the brief approach of his method and ensures that it is
engaged soon after he meets the patient for assessment.

Meandering through labyrinths and mandalas

Sacred and secular pilgrimages. Desoille's idea of moving in imaginative
space from top to bottom and from left to right echoes the walking pilgrims
in labyrinths. The paths intertwined by patient/pilgrim footsteps "weave"

the sacred and therapeutic spaces together. Pilgrimage is associated with the art of movement and the poetry of motion. The Medieval labyrinth has four quadrants that use the sacred geometry in its construction. This type is usually found on the floor of European churches such as Chartres Cathedral in France. During the Crusades when Christians could not make visits to the Holy Land, and the "Way of the Cross" devotion developed as a substitute pilgrimage to the Holy City, labyrinths came to be used as substitute of "*Chemins de Jerusalem*/Paths to Jerusalem."

A labyrinth has a well-defined path that weaves its way to the centre and back out again. For millennia, the labyrinth has been used by people across the world much like a mandala (Eliade, 1954). Labyrinths as mandalas have been used as spiritual journeys through the use of their sacred circles to the centre within them. Circularity is an important notion in psychotherapy. Circular motions around a centre and up and down movements are also common in dreams. One must make the circuit of one's complexes over and over again in the course of transformation. The alchemists referred to this stage as *circulatio* (Edinger, 1985). Jung himself speaks about labyrinths in conjunction with the process of analysis which leaves the person no choice but to face her- or himself. Furthermore, Jung like Eliade (1954) also juxtaposes the labyrinth with a mandala, from the labyrinth as a symbol that holds tension between order and chaos, to the mandala as an image of order itself. Jung eventually says that a mandala is the hallmark symbol of individuation and an "archetype of wholeness" (Jung, 1955/1968, p. 388 [CW9i, para. 715]).

As in a waking dream, one plans the journey, does the journey and walks back again. Actual pilgrimages, or labyrinth pilgrimages, as well as inner journeys, are capable of evoking emotions of awe, grief, reverence and joy. At such moments the patient/pilgrim crosses a threshold, a temporal emergence into eternal time and space whose properties infuse one's entire being. The landscape of difficulty and its perilous journey have always figured prominently in literature, from Gilgamesh to the Odyssey, and the temptation to remain in a safe environment is much eschewed by these heroes. George Bernard Shaw (1904) sees moral geography as a product of the Judeo-Christian civilisation which depicts the world as a "moral gymnasium." This idea though, played in an interior space, is strongly felt both in Jung and Desoille's accounts of their patient's waking dreams. Desoille, in coming up with a method of moving in a directed internal space,[6] has interiorised even further the idea of pilgrimage. Likewise, the same can be said of Jung's own exercises with mandala paintings, and his encouragement of his patients to paint their own.

Spaces of encounter in fantasy literature

The organs which habitually allow us to engage the world of concrete reality paradoxically also provide us with a space of encounter in waking dreams. A closer look at the nature of the figures encountered in active imagination and in the directed waking dream reveals that the fantasy figures are not the same. This is even more so if one had to analyse them from a fantasy literature[7] genre perspective. So far, there has been hardly any study of Jung's (2009) *The Red Book* and Desoille's approach in terms of their fantasy literary aspects. There have been several writings on *The Red Book*'s art style and value (Wojtkowski, 2009; Hale, 2010; Brutsche, 2011, Thackery, 2014; Mellick, 2018) which seem to have over-shadowed a focus on its literary style with the exception of Slattery (2011), which compares Jung's *The Red Book* in the epic poetry genre, for example Dante's *Divine Comedy*, and Rowland's (2013) understanding of active imagination as a close reading of text.

On one hand, in the case of active imagination, Jung stated in *Memories, Dreams, Reflections* that "no fantasy, none of the numerous images, no figure, could be traced back to personal biographical events" (Jung, 1963/1995, p. 66). While on the other for Desoille, every experience is uncanny in a Freudian sense, and many harrowing figures eventually are transformed in known figures from the patient's life. Furthermore, in the case of Desoille's RED method, the initial fantastic material encountered in the first waking dream sessions resembles more the characters found in a folktale, where the protagonist goes through several fantastic adventures aided by magic helpers.

In the Desoillian imaginative landscape, there is an ongoing shift and transformation of scenery, objects and people, who seem to dominate more than the dialogue with the characters, which is more prominent in Jung's (2009) *The Red Book*. However, in the case of Jung, he somehow distances himself from the realm of magic and seems to have been more influenced by ghost stories and spiritism in his writings of *The Red Book*, especially in the *Scrutinies*. Nonetheless, elements of magical thinking such as in the case of the death and resurrection of Izdubar and Jung's description of a fairy tale towards the end of *Liber Secundus* can be found, but seem to be rather less pronounced than in the Desoillian waking dream.

Post-Enlightenment philosophers and scientists claimed to have had the power to banish superstition; however, the attraction of folk metaphysics persisted in both rural and urban contexts and was reflected in the fantasy literature of Victorian and Edwardian periods. While folklorists collected legends from the rural working class, the educated elite engaged in spiritualist activities, from their supposed encounters with ghostly apparitions. The educated elite in Victorian and Edwardian periods wanted to be both mystical and scientific as is characteristic of their supernatural fiction writings (Harris, 2008).

In comparing Jung and Desoille's fantasy writing styles, one can also notice a subtle reference to their social class status. Jung prefers, maybe unconsciously, to adopt an elite way of writing about the supernatural, while Desoille chooses a more popular literary fantasy style. One can surely argue that this is just a matter of style, or that Jung and Desoille were writing with a certain audience in mind. However, this is rather strange in Jung's case since in *The Red Book* he tries to get in touch with himself by distancing himself from the wordly expectations such as ambition and wealth.

Both Desoille and Jung's accounts of waking dreams seem to fit with Rosemary Jackson's (1981) definition of fantasy. For Jackson, fantasy attempts to compensate for a lack resulting from "cultural constraint." When Jackson refers to "cultural constraint," she is referring to the oppressive power of "capitalist and patriarchal order" (Jackson, 1981, p. 76) and "bourgeois ideals" (ibid., p. 5), which fantasy literature militates against by showing the resistance of the unconscious mind to those laws. Jung had sacrificed his sonship to Freud by pursuing his own theories and was disappointed with the rationalistic era he was living in. Likewise, Desoille moved away from his mentor Eugene Caslant and was very disillusioned with the ravages of both the First and Second World Wars, as well as his loss of his first wife, Lucie (Eliade, 1973/1990). In some ways, in resorting to their own internal fantasy world, both Jung and Desoille tried to undo their personal losses as well as to address the moral deficit in the Western world's balance sheet. For the American playwright Tennessee William, the writers in the "long weekend" between the wars tried to compensate for the malaise of place loss by throwing themselves into motion, and in the words of the protagonist Tom in Williams' *Glass Menagerie* they attempted "to find in motion what was lost in space" (Williams, 1945, p. 75).

Jung's encounter with fantasy figures, be they mythological or purely fantastical, are described with fear and trepidation, and he greets them with suspicion. Furthermore, he is aware of their autonomous existence which at times can manifest physically through the psychoid level. For Jung, in active imagination one moves outside linear movement of time to the acausal, non-deterministic dimension. Jung's attitude evokes Tzvetan Todorov's (1975) idea of the marvellous fantasy, i.e., the truly supernatural, while in the case of Desoille, it is more a case of uncanny fantasy encounters, even though their effect on the patient's psyche is very much felt. For Todorov, uncanny fantasy is explainable by recourse to existing laws of nature and should not be confused with marvellous fantasy that denotes events or people that are disquieting and mysterious.

Private affairs in public spaces

While Jung and Desoille chose different ways to move inside their waking dream approaches, both of them insisted on the need to give some form of flesh to the images either through writing, painting, or using other creative media. One striking difference is that in Desoille's directed waking dream, the therapist is actually present and listens *in vivo* to the narrative of the unfolding oneiro-dramatic performance of the patient. Jung, when practising active imagination, chooses to remain alone, away from the eyes of the other.

There is something of an oral cult in Desoille's waking dream. The French theorist Michel de Certeau (1984) used the term "spatial stories" in *The Practice of Everyday Life* to emphasise the interdependency of textual narratives and spatial practices. He speaks of a "walking rhetoric" (ibid., p. 97), i.e., a close relationship between walking and talking. The Desoillian therapist acts like a witness and a biographer of the patient's *itinerarium intus* as the patient transforms the inside into an outside by means of the art of telling. Through the patient's direct verbal account of his or her inner experience, the patient fulfils a need to tell his or her story, something which the active imagination as practised by Jung and classic Jungians does not offer. One value of vivid, detailed description lies in prompting linear thinking while employing nonlinear thinking at the same time, thus achieving a balance of these two activities. The RED therapist like a religious mystic biographer, usually the spiritual director, keeps notes of the patient/mystic's progress. The therapist like the spiritual director makes the oracle-like subject speak. The director makes audible the subject's voice and thus follows the ancient maxim *Loquere ut te Videam*, i.e., speak so that I may see you. Piny's request to Socrates to disclose himself combines the verbal and the visual (Paige, 2001). In so doing, the RED therapist engages in a hermeneutic of suspicion since he can later check his written recorded version with that of the patient's recollections and reveal any blind spots. Therefore, in the directed waking dream, the patient's words are not necessarily the Bible truth. It seems that one's inner truths can be expressed and written only with difficulty, even though RED caters for a disinhibition effect. Echoing the psychoanalyst Masud Khan's views on Winnicott, RED "also creates a secret space in the area of note-taking that matches the patient's secret space in couch-sleep. Thus, both are safe with each other and survive each other" (Khan, 1986, p. 18). The interior is that which escapes. It is also assumed that like the power of the religious biography to move the reader, the patient and therapist's written accounts influence and help them in the process of mutual transformation. Nonetheless, the issue of making public one's secrets is not all positive. Jung himself in his later life did voice some of his memories of his waking dreams to his secretary, Aniele Jaffe, who acted almost like a RED therapist, which eventually became a chapter in *Memories, Dreams, Reflections* (1963). However, the controversies of the politics of editions is public history (Shamdasani, 1995). In 2009, Jung's family heirs did agree to publish *The Red Book* once they felt that very little harm could be done to Jungian psychoanalysis, something which Jung was very much afraid of, especially from the scientific community. Jung's fears of being "indexed," echo the mystics' caution of what to say to biographers, or how much to write in their autobiographies. Issues of external power limit how much self-disclosure can be allowed. Jung's (2009) *The*

Red Book attests to the depths of his soul. However, his drawings seem to interest us more than his dialogues since they convey more of the unsaid. Total secrecy seems to be as impossible as total exposure.

Notes

1 The journey theme is one of the great archetypal themes of world literature. Great epics such as *The Odyssey*, *The Aeneid* and *The Ramayana* present the adventures of a hero who sets out on a journey. The collective journey of the Hebrew people in the exodus constitutes the central spiritual experience of the Judaic tradition. The journey of the soul to the Good is the central theme of Plotinus' *Enneads*. The inner spiritual journey of Dante in the *Divine Comedy* stands as one of the greatest poetic and religious expression of Western civilisation. From Gilgamesh to Frodo of The Lord of the Rings, the quest and search is a fundamental theme of humanity. To be human is to be *homo viator*. The outer quest may be more Western, the inner quest more Eastern.

2 Postmodernism is a philosophical movement which is largely a reaction against the philosophical assumptions and values of the modern period of Western (specifically European) history, i.e., the period from about the time of the scientific revolution of the sixteenth and seventeenth centuries to the mid-twentieth century. Indeed, many of the doctrines characteristically associated with postmodernism can fairly be described as the straightforward denial of general philosophical viewpoints or metanarratives that were taken for granted during the modern period. For a critical study of postmodernism, see *Post-Modern Theory: Critical Interrogations* by S. Best and D. Kellner (1991) and *Postmodernism: A Very Short Introduction* by C. Butler (2003).

3 "The shadow," wrote Jung (1963), is "that hidden, repressed, for the most part inferior and guilt-laden personality whose ultimate ramifications reach back into the realm of our animal ancestors and so comprise the whole historical aspect of the unconscious" (CW 9ii, para. 422). Jung differentiated between the *personal shadow* and the impersonal or *archetypal shadow*, which acknowledges transpersonal, pure or radical evil (symbolised by the Devil and demons) and collective evil.

4 Raphael's painting of the *Transfiguration* also epitomises this process. It is a common mythological motif that a human is taken up to heaven to meet the angels and even God himself.

5 It refers to a psychic function that arises from the tension between the consciousness and the unconscious and supports their union. Jung defines it in his essay *The Transcendent Function* as "The tendencies of the conscious and the unconscious are the two factors that together make up the transcendent function. It is called 'transcendent' because it makes the transition from one attitude to another organically possible" (CW 8, para. 145).

6 Desoille's interiorisation of wandering in imaginative space echoes the Rousseaun tradition of "*Les Rêveries du Promeneur Solitaire*/The Reveries of a Solitary Walker," i.e., walking as a state of self-reflection and reverie. Moreover, the French poet Arthur Rimbaud was to coin the verb *robinsonner* (meaning to travel mentally) in recognition of this very activity, and it becomes increasingly difficult to distinguish between the figure of the flaneur and the mental or stationary traveller.

7 Fantasy is a genre of fiction that uses magic or other supernatural elements as a main plot element, theme or setting. Many works within the genre take place in imaginary worlds where magic and magical creatures are common.

Chapter 12

Conceptualising a theoretical comparison of RED and active imagination

After having compared the two waking dream methods based on spatial metaphors of interiority, this chapter attempts a broader theoretical comparison between the procedural aspects of both RED and active imagination. Categories to organise the comparison are established from the Jungian and Desoillian literature review which are common to both approaches, although their emphasis in each approach differs. The categories are setting and preparation of the body, structure and directivity by the analyst/therapist, transferential and counter-transferential relationship, narratives and interpretation. The comparison which is built on different categories will help us identify commonalities and divergences between RED and active imagination. On a general level, the main ideas of RED that are in accordance with the principles of active imagination are that it stops the dangers of free-flowing fantasising, RED provides a clearer language than dreams do, and a more immediate and involving personal experience of unconscious processes. Furthermore, it helps to develop a capacity to imagine, have a symbolic attitude, and is easier than active imagination because of its more or less established setting and relative guidance by the therapist. RED not only bridges the gap between inner and outer worlds, but also seems to fit well with different theoretical positions including analytical psychology. Based on the comparative study of the two approaches, I will then explore the implications for a "hybridised" and integrative clinical practice framework of a RED-based approach to active imagination. I will attempt to stay with the tension of holding an appreciation as well as an assimilation of differences in RED and active imagination.

Integrative perspective

"Integration" refers to a general flexible and inclusive attitude towards different psychotherapeutic models (Greben, 2004). It aims to see what can be learned and introduced from various perspectives in practice. An integrative approach advocates for a systematic process to develop a conceptual framework that includes ways to select theories and techniques that are compatible (Jensen, Bergin & Greaves, 1990; Lapworth & Sills, 2010). Integration in psychotherapy involves four possible approaches, all of which are, to a certain extent, in play in the current project to develop a RED-based approach to active imagination:

1   Theoretical integration (i.e., transcending diverse models by creating a single but different approach).
2   Technical eclecticism (i.e., using effective ingredients from different approaches).
3   Common factors approach (i.e., focusing on effective therapeutic practices that are common to all approaches).
4   Assimilative integration approach (i.e., the gradual process of incorporating attitudes, perspectives, ideas or techniques from other therapies and assimilating these into one's own main theoretical framework).

In addition to the four paradigms, there is a fifth route: a pluralistic approach, which is becoming increasingly influential in meeting the current challenges in the field. O'Hara and Schofield (2008) consider that pluralism is one approach to manage the tension created by the use of different theories. Adopting a pluralistic approach enables therapists to use a variety of theories without the need to reconcile differences. The pluralistic view is postmodernist insofar as truth is seen as constructed more than discovered, where the philosophy underpinning it holds that "any substantial question admits of a variety of plausible but mutually conflicting responses" (Cooper & McLeod, 2007, p. 137). Samuels describes pluralism as "an attitude to conflict which tries to reconcile differences without imposing a false resolution on them or losing sight of the unique value of each position. As an ideology, pluralism seeks to hold unity and diversity in balance [....]" (Samuels, 1989, p. 33).

Assimilative integration

Despite the earlier statement that all the existing approaches to psychotherapy integration are being held in mind, there is no doubt that the most useful is assimilative integration. I have used an assimilative integration approach to develop the framework of a RED-based active imagination. After doing the comparative work between the two approaches, I will explore ways to fit aspects of RED which are theoretically aligned to active imagination and are coherent with the principles of analytical psychology. As a result, I will be adopting a contextualist position (Pepper, 1942) in which a therapeutic technique is viewed, not as standing on its own, but deriving its meaning from the theory or therapy in which it is employed. Furthermore, we have also seen that several Jungian analysts (Garufi, 1977; Plateo Zoja, 1978; Kast, 1998, Kroke, 2004) have argued for adapting active imagination to the therapy session, especially when patients find it hard to engage with symbolic material and would need to be guided in how to do this. RED offers this to patients.

Assimilative integration is the practice of absorbing a technique or idea from one therapy approach into the main theory within which one is grounded, with the imported technique influenced by the context into which it is absorbed (Messer, 2001). Assimilative integration is believed to be an inevitable part of the development of most psychotherapists. It involves the smooth flow of one technique into another, rather than an inelegant or sudden introduction of an intervention, which might seem strange or inappropriate to a client. A technique cannot stand alone and separate from the therapy within which it is practised (ibid.). Lampropoulos (2001) and Downing (2004) believe assimilative integration is the combination of theoretical integration and technical eclecticism and achieved in such a way that may reconcile some of their conflicts. If eclecticisim and integration are regarded as existing on a continuum, assimilative integration can be located somewhere mid-way. It compensates for the pull between the focus on techniques in eclectisim and an emphasis on a conceptual framework in integrationism (Downing, 2004).

Lampropoulos refers to assimilative integration as a mini-theoretical integration. Carere-Comes (2001) believes that assimilative integration is interchangeable with theoretical integration. The overlap with theoretical integration is evident in the assimilative approach because there has to be at least a modest consilience between the ethos of the theoretical home base and the rationale of the technique that is assimilated into it. An assimilative position which favours a firm grounding in any one system of psychotherapy does not necessarily exclude any or all accommodative modifications (Strickler & Gold, 1996). It is true that if a process is defined as assimilative, it is because assimilation prevails over accommodation but prevalence does not mean exclusion of the necessary counterpart.

Assimilative integration leads to enrichment of the field and to pluralism. This approach can be seen as falling within a "pluralistic tradition, which holds that one theory or model can never pre-empt or preclude an alternate organisation of the evidence" (Norcross & Goldfried, 2005, p. 2). This stance contends that we need several theories of therapy at any one time, because the best way of achieving the most appropriate solution is through the ongoing challenging of multiple competing theories with each other and with the evidence (Messer, 2001).

Hybridity

An integrated RED-based approach to active imagination is aimed at ending years of misunderstanding about working with imagery, and at times hostility between the two imaginative approaches. The two waking dream

approaches, i.e., RED and active imagination, might have seemed irrec-
oncilable for a long time. This chapter aims to move away from a climate
of factionalism and parochialism between schools and towards dialogue
and rapproachement. This hovering between two waking dream methods
evokes Hermes and his tricksterish qualities which initiate us into seeing
things in different ways while challenging at times rigid and privileged Jungian perceptions. Thus, I will explore RED's contribution to active imagination by carving out a new space, where the two methods can possibly
meet. I will attempt to hold the tension between an appreciation and an
assimilation of differences in RED and active imagination. As a result of
this comparison, an integrated hybridised clinical practice framework will
emerge, possibly leading to a better understanding of the use of active imagination in the therapy itself.

Hybridity refers in its most basic sense to mixture. The term originates
from biology and was subsequently employed in linguistics and racial theory in the nineteenth century (Young, 1995). Its contemporary uses are
found across numerous academic disciplines, as well as in popular culture.
The term carries opposing connotations. On one hand, it is celebrated given
its association with the richness of syncretism, and, on the other hand,
it spells fears of "contamination" to those who espouse essentialist and
purist perspectives (Kraidy, 2005). In psychotherapy, it refers to a process
of using various practical and theoretical elements of different therapeutic
approaches and blends them together to create a new brand therapy approach (often acronymic in title). The "pharmacopoeia" of psychotherapy
is vast. Garfield and Bergin (1994) claim that there are over 400 varieties
of therapy.

The RED-based approach to active imagination will be different from
the RED method andactive imagination but will include elements from
both. The RED-based approach to active imagination will be developed
through the analysis of each category, used for the comparative study, both
from a Desoillian and Jungian perspective. The rationale of how elements
and ideas from RED consistent with principles in analytical psychology
can possibly be integrated in the practice of active imagination will be
provided. The emphasis in this thesis is on integration, a term which is more
commonly used when bridging theoretical therapeutic ideas. However, hybridity, which is usually used to refer to final distinct clinical psychotherapeutic models, is here used in conjunction with the term integrated, i.e., in
the phrase "hybridised-integrated" approach, in order to add flavour and
definition. In the next chapters, the key propositions and concepts chosen for a RED-based approach to active imagination which make up the
hybridised- integrated approach will be highlighted, grouped and presented
as a practice framework for clinicians using directed waking dreams. This
framework can be developed further into a full hybrid clinical therapeutic
model in the future.

Chapter 13

A theoretical comparison of RED and active imagination

Getting started preparation of the body and directivity by the analyst

In this and the next chapter, the two therapeutic approaches will be compared using the following five categories, namely: setting and preparation of the body, structure and directivity by the analyst/therapist, transferential and counter-transferential relationship, narratives and interpretation. This comparison will help to identify commonalities and divergences between RED and active imagination. This chapter compares the two approaches from the point of view of the first two categories listed above, i.e., setting and preparation of the body, and structure and directivity by the therapist which have to do with the initial stages of the therapeutic process.

Body therapy on the couch

The use of body work is found in different theoretical psychotherapeutic models. In fact, psychotherapy can be situated along a continuum from verbal to non-verbal. There are verbal psychotherapies that give little or no attention to the body that are situated on one side of the continuum. Nonetheless in therapy, therapists and patients are not just "talking," but also "bodies interacting." Moving further on the continuum, we find approaches working with a different aspect of the body, such as paying attention to non-verbals or somatic counter-transference, to fully formalised and systematised techniques. These can be used as a treatment by themselves like, for example, "Bioenergetics" or "Hakomi." Totton (2003) identifies three models in body psychotherapy: the adjustment model, the trauma/discharge model and the process oriented model. The adjustment model sees therapy as a corrective experience that re-aligns the body and thus the mind. The discharge model emphasises emotional expression in a safe space, while the process model sees the therapist as a guide to the patient in the journey and brings the therapeutic emphasis much more into the present moment. Several body therapies integrate more than one of these models in their approach. These models can also help us to better locate the use of the body in RED and active imagination.

The body in RED

Desoille in his RED method retained the lying down position, a remnant of hypnosis, and worked in a semi-obscure therapy setting where he sat behind the patient. He also underlined the importance of relaxing the body; if people had difficulties unwinding, they needed to be sent to a separate person for autogenic training relaxation (Desoille, 1973). According to Desoille, a relaxed position and a semi-dark therapy setting led one to imagine more effectively.

For Desoille, and even more so for his disciple Dr. Marc Guillery, the development of an imaginal ego,[1] which interacted in the imaginative landscape through all the senses in the waking dream, seemed to be more relevant than the actual body itself. The focus was on the embodied representation of oneself in the waking dream. In fact, problems related to an inability to imagine the self could be indicative of resistance. Some patients could have difficulty seeing their faces in imagery. Some could only see their backs. Often this indicated a resistance to feelings of shame and guilt. Desoille (1938) himself spoke about the difficulties of neurasthenic patients to engage in waking dreams since many times their images were pale and lacked energy. Furthermore, Desoille was particularly interested in the patients' feelings in the waking dream. Desoille realised that images may uncover intense affective states or elicit emotional reactions.[2] In moments of anxiety, patients tend to move or hold themselves. Therefore, the recumbent body still manages to convey a lot to the therapist, even though the person is lying down.

Desoille also realised from his research in 1938 that the waking dream is capable of producing very diverse physiological changes in the body, a finding that followed the teachings of the Indian yogi master Swami Siddheswarananda[3] who was in France at that time (Choisy, 1949). Numerous studies after Desoille have corroborated his findings (Barber, 1961, 1965; Simpson & Paivio, 1966; Achterberg, 1984; Kunzendorf & Sheikh, 1990). Nonetheless, Desoille could not escape the powerful influence of Cartesian dualism: he limited his waking dream method to the treatment of the so-called psychological problems and did not apply it to physical ones while still believing that physiological changes in the body were a secondary derivative of the waking dream.

Historically, the use of the imagination in psychotherapy developed from two routes. One has been through the introspective school, associated with Binet who later influenced Happich and Kretschmer. They believed that images arising in introspection expressed different sub-personalities of the patient. However, another group of researchers arrived at similar uses of waking dreams, "not through the practise of introspection [...] but through a bio-physical approach to consciousness" (Watkins, 1976, p. 55). J.H. Schultz, influenced by Vogt's work on auto-hypnotic exercises, realised that a hypnotic state could occur if the patient could suggest to self that he or she was having feelings of warmth and heaviness which, in turn, would lead to a relaxed state. Meditative exercises were also given once an "autogenic" relaxed stage was reached that included visualisations and waking dreams. Frank's (1910) "catarthic method" and Guillerey's "*rêve vecu*/lived dream" (1955) also emphasised the importance of physiology in waking dreams.

Another colleague of Desoille, Andre Virel, also started the imaginative process by giving importance to the physiological process of the body. Virel gave special importance to sensation of the body in his "*decentration/ de-centring*" technique, as part of his "*oneirotherapie d'integration/*onei-rotherapy of integration" (1970–1971). He did not want to silence the body by relaxation (thus the name *decentration*). Virel would ask the patient to focus on his or her body and be aware of sensations (especially in the finger tips) and images in the first stages of therapy with the aim of disengaging from the usual perception of one's body so as to recreate a new bodily sense, a new "*scheme corporel*/body scheme." This loosening up of the body image facilitates changes to one's psychic attitude.

The body in active imagination

In contrast to Desoille, Jung seemed to give less importance to the preparation of the body. In *Yoga and the West*, Jung stated that the method of active imagination consisted in a "special training for switching off consciousness" (Jung, 1936/1969, pp. 536–537 [CW11, para. 875]) but he did not specify what this training is. However, Jung chose not to emphasise the body element in preparation for active imagination despite being *au courant* of the "Autogenic training" of Schultz (1932/1958) and Freud's initial so-called "pressure technique" (1895), which involved lightly touching the hand of the patient so they would be better able to free associate through images. Jung was also aware of the preparation of the physical body in Loyola's Spiritual Exercises and in Eastern meditation practices.

Nonetheless, Jung at one point, during his own experiences of active imagination, described how he had to resort to "certain yoga exercises," without going in detail as to what they were, to "hold his emotions in check" (Jung, 1963/1995, p. 201). This shows the importance of grounding oneself in the body before engaging in imaginative work since as Jung has emphasised, active imagination is very serious play. It could very well be that Jung, despite knowing the importance of preparing the body, may have wanted to move away from these known body approaches and may not have wanted to risk coming up with a method which would be so similar to other known approaches in his time.

There is no doubt that Jung believed in the mind-body connection and that they were "two sides of the same coin, and [that] [...] this whole separation of mind [is] [...] merely a device of reason for the purpose of conscious discrimination" (Jung, 1926/1960, p. 326 [CW8, para. 619]). Through his word association experiments in the early 1900s, Jung discovered that the complex has a feeling tone aspect to it and is associated with physiological reactions, with the processes of the heart, the tonus of the blood vessels, the condition of the intestines, the breathing and the innervation of the skin. Jung understood that images could be expressed and experienced through any or all of the sensory modalities of the body, i.e., the classic five senses, as well as through somato-sensory sensations including muscular, vestibular, visceral body reactions and body temperature.

Body implications for a RED-based active imagination

A RED-based approach of active visual imagination can integrate very well the idea of giving importance to the body both in preparing it before it starts the oneiric drama and in using the somato-sensory reactions of the body as stimuli for an imaginative experience. Both a couch and the armchair can be used; however, in the case of couch-work the therapist has to sit side-ways, in a way that he or she can be seen by the patient, unlike what happens in RED and psychoanalytic RED. The Jungian analyst, Verena Kast, when using "guided imaginings," prefers to work with an armchair so that the patient can have his or her feet well grounded on the floor, leading to "an additional containment, a grounding in the body" (Kast, 1993, p. 20). This view was also shared by Desoille's Algerian-Israeli disciple Colette Aboulkher-Muscat. Therefore, grounding can be both "vertical" and "horizontal" (Totton, 2003). However, research (Berdach & Bakan, 1967; Segal & Glicksman, 1967; Singer & Antrobus, 1972) has shown that when lying down, the imagery quality tends to improve. I think one has to check how the patient feels, since lying down with eyes closed in a semi-dark room may feel quite threatening.

The idea of starting active imagination from the body itself in the Jungian tradition is associated with "Authentic Movement therapy," founded by Mary Stark Whitehouse. Similar methods were also explored and developed by Jungian analyst Arnold Mindell (1985) in his "Process-oriented psychology." Mindell analyses the body's sensations and symptoms as if he is analysing a dream, calling it "dream body." The body dreams not only in the visual and auditory ways of experiencing in dream work, but also in the inner body feelings, movements and sensations. Nonetheless, patients with strong intuitive functions might resist focusing on sensations in the body and a simple relaxation exercise would probably be more appropriate for them. Imagination and moving in imaginative space evoke feelings, sensations, emotions and memory. The therapist can help connect the patient present to his or her imagination to an embodied here and now. Such an approach supports a psyche-soma integration. The somatic aspect of imagery is also emphasised in Dr. Ahsen's "Eidetic psychotherapy" (1965), which is built on a tripartite structure of image, somatic response and meaning (I.S.M.). Thus, a RED-based active imagination becomes an activity of seeing not only with our eyes but with our whole being, since vision is not the activity of a disembodied eye but a project of a human being situated in a place, time, culture and a body that is implicated in these contexts.

The clinical aspect of RED related to the concept of resistance in images of the body-self during the oneiro-drama can also be applied in active imagination, since the latter has remained more focused on the creative transformative aspect and does not describe strongly enough the manifestation of psychopathology during imagery. Active imagination can continue to benefit from looking at RED's clinical applications, which are more developed and further researched.

Structure and directivity

In contrast to Jungians who preferred to engage in active imagination alone or to remain witnesses while the method was being used in the therapy session itself, Desoille in his RED method broke the cardinal rule of neutrality and adopted directivity. His suggestions were aimed at helping to stimulate the imagination of the subject. Thus, Desoille brought a somewhat relational stance to the therapy. Desoille emphasised that in giving directions it is imperative that the therapist would have had his or her own therapeutic personal journey so as to know his or her own blind spots. RED centres on a dialectical interplay of self-expression and a gentle form of relational guidance and engagement.

From an analytical psychology perspective, the therapist's presence seems to take on the ego function of the patient in order to help the patient deal better with his or her images. This may in turn help the ego complex of the patient to separate from the parental complexes leading to a stronger ego identity. If we look at the function of the RED therapist on a continuum, on one end there is witnessing, while at the other end there is the guiding style, in which the therapist is quite participatory. The therapist attunes his style according to the needs of the patient. The therapist's role is minimal, becoming participatory, even directive, only if necessary. Directives centre around these elements: the giving of initial stimuli, encouragement to the patient to immerse himself or herself and explore oneiric space, to move up and down a vertical imaginative axis, and to imaginatively hold ground, and help the patient when faced with challenging and menacing figures or situations while engaged in an oneiric drama.

Stimuli

RED initial stimuli

A main characteristic of Desoille's RED is the giving of the initial stimulus which helps the patient develop a waking dream. The therapist does not suggest the whole fantasy but directs it by offering word stimuli which can serve as crystallisation for the waking dream. I prefer to call these initial stimuli *enargeic*[4] stimuli or inceptive cues which could be verbal, auditory, visual or kinaesthetic although the most commonly practised is verbal. The sensation of the stimulus in RED leads to a change in perception, accessing archaic memory, fantasies and repressed desires and firing a creative transformative imagination. The *enargeic* stimulus helps free the patient's imaginative experience leading to a *drame interieur*, involving an unfolding of what urgently seeks expression. The stimulus is a powerful and direct route into the imaginal and the way can lead downwards into hell and upwards into heaven.

The word stimuli are akin to magic words although their function is different to the ritual of "casting a spell." According to Malinowski, "the most important element in magic is the spell" (Malinowski, 1954, p. 132). Each culture will naturally have its own set of spells. The verbal stimuli act like a wand in the hand of the therapist. They can indicate focus as well as spark creative inspiration. The Desoillian initial stimuli remind us of Bachelard's description of certain nouns as "children of the night" (Bachelard, 1960, p. 35). Bachelard speaks of the temperament of words and that words "do not have the same psychic 'weight' depending on whether they belong to the language of reverie or to the language of daylight life" (ibid., p. 58). In fact, in post-Desoillian schools, different stimuli have been developed from the original six employed by Desoille and the art of the therapist lies in his or her ability to create and match the right stimulus to the right problem being faced. The shadow side of the wand, however, is associated with control and power when the therapist becomes too directive, when the situation calls for patience and staying with uncertainty. Post-Desoillians today, especially those of a psychoanalytic orientation, seem to have done away with giving structured stimuli, but rely on "ego-syntonic" stimuli, i.e., that are derived directly from the patient's repertoire, as in the practice of active imagination. Another starting point is through the use of psychological tests or projective tests where words or images can be used as stimuli to the patient. Incidentally, Desoille (1945) himself has seen the close similarity between his *image de depart* and the word association test of Carl Jung. Jung's work on the word association experiment connects words with unconscious processes, which produce affects revealed in complex indicators. However, there is no evidence that Desoille or post-Desoillians have used Jung's test as an *image de depart* in therapy.

The therapist is important not only as a hearing audience, a beholder, but as a body and a presence. The therapist can also choose to share some of his or her counter-transference in the form of a stimulus on which the patient can engage in an oneiro-drama. This technique has been developed by post-Desoillians from the psychoanalytic camp where the waking dream itself is a third pole arising in between the pole of the analyst and the other pole of the patient. This post-Desoillian development runs parallel to the Jungian idea of the intermediate space between patient and analyst which arises in the therapeutic relationship (Schwartz-Salant, 1986; Samuels, 1989) and Corbin's idea of the *Mundus Imaginalis* (1972).

The non-prescriptiveness of active imagination

To the contrary, Jung remains decidedly non-prescriptive about the images of active imagination, leaving them up to each patient's invention. In the *Visions Seminars* (1930–1934), Jung said that "Everybody wants to have his way prescribed so that he has not to bother with it" (Jung, 1998, p. 888). Jung's strategy to confront one's unconscious is a demanding one, since it requires the patient's concentration to give birth to the pure image in perfect solitude. One cannot borrow it from external sources, one must create it. Jung presumed the soul itself is the source of its own symbols that best express what is going on intra-psychically.

Jung in fact objected that the spiritual exercises of Loyola and other systems of spirituality can cripple a process of active imagination by confining it to predetermined images. Jung was critical of these spiritual exercises since the goal must be reached in the prescribed time with the tremendous effort of the will. Jung prefers the practice of the *Devotio Moderna*,[5] who submerged themselves in God to reach inner peace. Moreover, "[...] the path of the *Devoti* led inwards, that of Ignatius outwards: deeds, battle, enterprise attacks on the world, the right use of will were the goal. Mysticism was dissolved in a method" (Jung, 1939–1940, p. 173).

Jung was also against the use of drugs to alter the states of consciousness such as mescaline, which he had learnt about from Dr. Prinzhorn, since with drugs one could manipulate the brain so that it produces even so-called "spiritual" experiences. In a letter to Christian Stamm in 1949, Jung affirmed that there is no need "to try and loosen up the unconscious." However, he gave an exception when he said "though an honest drink would none forbid" had been regarded as "sacrosanct" from a very long time (Jung, 1973, p. xiv).

Implications of the use of stimuli in a RED-based active imagination

Although it is more controversial for the therapist from a classic Jungian perspective to introduce external stimuli in the session, one can argue that in the initial stages of therapy it might be useful if patients did not report dream material. Jungians can present to the patient stimuli from the patient's own material or else give them ones related to the main Jungian concepts such as shadow, anima or animus, as well as from mythology and fairy tales, as well as Tarot cards, which are so frequently studied by Jungi-ans. In the *Transcendent Function*, Jung (1916/1960) observed:

> we find cases where there is no tangible mood or depression at all, but just a general dull discontent, a feeling of resistance to everything, a sort of boredom or vague disgust, an indefinable but excruciating emp-tiness. In these cases no definite starting point exists – it would first have to be created.
>
> (Jung, 1958/1960, p. 83 [CW8, para. 169])

RED in contrast to Jung's active imagination offers a different and more benevolent kind of descent into that nether realm, unlike the myth of Persephone and her abduction by Hades into the underworld. As Down-ing (1993) observes, the reflection of Hermes' role as psychopomp leads us to think about the underworld experience in a particular way, and his approach is one of being guided to rather than abducted to the underworld. This experience of being guided to access unconscious roots of one's com-plexes can be seen by the practices of some Jungians. For example, in the book *Encounters with the Soul – Active Imagination as Developed by C.G. Jung*, Barbara Hannah speaks about her patient, Anna Marjula, who she eventually referred to Emma Jung. Hannah reported that the active imagination her patient was undergoing was not working and Emma pre-scribed to her the idea of engaging in a dialogue with "some positive female archetype such as the Great Mother" (Hannah, 1981, p. 138) in her active imagination, a suggestion which proved to be successful.

In sand play therapy, the objects on display which children or adults use to put in the sand tray are also a form of stimuli. Turner (2005) states that she groups her sand tray figures in two ways: by developmental level and then by archetype. An example of developmental grouping is the place-ment of the items on a shelf that a child may choose, corresponding to the child's height. Regarding archetypal grouping, Turner (2005) places all of the earthly elements, such as rocks and earthly items on the ground, and religious figures on higher shelves. Furthermore, the "intensive journal method" of Jungian analyst Ira Progoff (1975) is a structured one and is categorised into sections, such as the time/life dimension, daily log and dream states, and offers self-dialogue sections for the body, work, persons, events, society and one's inner wisdom states.

Since the RED method shows a good ability to stimulate the deeper lev-els of the unconscious and to do it quickly, one has to show caution when making use of it. In fact, one has to remain careful not to lose the focus on analytic work where the therapist is a servant of psyche and not a healer (Lopez-Pedroza, 1977), especially when proposing different suggestive words to bypass resistance or to influence the unconscious mind. The latter became more pronounced in RED when Desoille became influenced with Milton Erickson's[6] work on hypnosis in his later career.

The issue of when to introduce stimuli into the session is also worth pondering. It is important that the introduction of stimuli, so as to try out oneiric dramas with patients, has to happen gradually after a good history of the patient where testing has been done. The patient can also be assessed in regard to his or her ability to benefit from imaginative techniques. This can be done by carrying out a short exercise to test the patient's ability to visualise through a simple test, such as trying to imagine an object, such as a flower. The introduction and the type of stimuli used could also be done from metaphors the patient uses, such as "I feel like I am in a narrow alley right now in my life," and then the therapist can ask the patient to continue this trope in fantasy. Although a spontaneous stimulus should be preferred over a suggested one by the therapist, sometimes, a chosen one can cause the patient to emotionally contact certain issues he or she might be avoiding. My hypothesis is in line with the research of Horowitz and Becker (1971), who state that the use of stimuli for visual imagery increases the tendency to form, as well as to report, images. Another alternative can be to start fantasies related to the keywords from the word association test or other projective tests that indicate the patient's complexes, thus ensuring continuity to the therapeutic work. A case in point is Leuner's "guided affective imagery" method which is divided in the psychodiagnostic phase and in the therapeutic phase (Leuner, 1969). The first part, i.e., the psychodiagnostic phase, is known as "initiated symbol projection." In it, the ten initial stimuli employed are used as projective stimuli as in a projective psychological test such as the "Thematic Apperception Test." Only a limited response to each of the presented stimuli is allowed in the first phase, which is akin to Jung's word association test. The answers are later explored in more depth in the second stage of the method.

Imaginative movement: spontaneous vs. directed movement

One of the main characteristics of images in our psyche is that they are autonomous, they have a life of their own. Yet, images are still under the control of the one engaged in an imaginative experience: both therapist and patient can manipulate the images in terms of setting and process. The extent of intervention both by the therapist and by the patient is one of the main ideas that distinguish RED from active imagination.

RED: on moving and being moved

In RED, patients become inner pilgrims since if "pilgrimage may be thought of as extroverted mysticism, [...] mysticism is introverted pilgrimage. The pilgrim physically traverses a mystical way; the mystic sets forth on an interior spiritual pilgrimage" (Turner, 1978, pp. 33–34). Instead of spiritual transformation, RED looks at an emotional metamorphosis. RED, much like Jung's analytical psychology, helps the patient through his or her impasse, towards a personal evolution and transformation, since the aim of the therapy is not an exploration of the past, as in psychoanalysis. Desoille would help the patients by stimulating their imagination and never by imposing his will on them. Besides a movement towards the future, RED underlines the importance of moving beyond the ordinary states of consciousness towards a higher spiritual level as well as a synthesis of opposites. Ascension and sublimation are the hallmarks of RED, achieved through movement in oneiric space around the vertical axis. Prof. Mario Berta (2000), an Uruguayan disciple of Desoille, states that personal maturity occurs in three directions:

'en avant' (anticipation), 'en haut' (ascenscion) et 'a cote' (polarisation). L'evolution existentielle est ainsi un processus complexe qui implique le fait simultane' d'anticiper le future par des anticipations precises, de 'monter; vers les niveaux surordonnes de conscience et de polariser les oppositions caracteristiques du monde dans lequel vit l'etre humain.

forward (anticipation); above (ascension) and sideways (polarisation). The existential evolution is a rather complex process which implies the simultaneous anticipation of the future with precise anticipations, of rising towards higher levels of consciousness and a polarisation of opposing characteristics of the world in which man lives.

(Berta, 2000, p. 12 [my translation])

Desoille's borrowing of Jung's ideas of archetypal images from the collective unconscious (1945) explained how during several waking dreams, the images tend to move from those encountered in normal dreams, to images related to folklore and myths, and finally to images of light and transcendence as therapy progresses. Desoille also believed that in facing the heights, the patient can sublimate his or her emotions, which are reflected in the figures encountered. Desoille further explained that the reintegration of the conflicting images into their archetypal series helps to achieve a synthesis of the psyche and fulfil its "function regulatrice/regulatory function" (Desoille, 1945, p. 325). Given the anxiety which is triggered in facing the depths, Desoille was very cautious not to encourage exploration of the lower aspects from the beginning implicating that the heights are less anxiety-provoking.

Spontaneous movement in active imagination

For Jung, spirit is the dynamic principle made up of:

[...] firstly, the principle of spontaneous movement and activity; secondly, the spontaneous capacity to produce images independently of sense perception; and thirdly, the autonomous and sovereign manipulation of these images.

(Jung, 1948/1968, p. 212 [CW9i, para. 393])

For Jung, psychic energy moves throughout the space of the psyche and does the work of the personality. Jung used the terms "libido" and "energy" interchangeably. Fundamental to energy in the psyche is movement which depends upon the principle of opposites. Although energy moves in many directions, Jung focused on progression and regression. When the psyche is balanced and energy flows out to life creatively, the libido is said to be in a progressive movement from the unconscious to conscious life. When psychic balance breaks, regression ensues and the energy begins to move deeper into the psyche. Regression is a return to the psyche so that the progressive movement of adaptation to the outer world may continue.

Classical Jungians not only do not introduce any external images to reflect on, but also prefer to stay with the images and let nature work "without our obnoxious intervention" (Jung, 1998, p. 393). Jung (1929/1967) referred to this meditative part in terms of *wu vei*, that is, the Taoist idea of letting things happen. Jung used to encourage practitioners of this method to observe the scene in a special attentive way known as *betrachten*, until things move spontaneously, rather than to consciously fill the scene with one's desired changes. Jung was also aware that when the ego enters into an active imagination, it is bound to be faced with endless and chaotic shifting which can cause the ego to get confused and lost. For Jung, every archetype can reveal itself in a plurality of possible manifestations as it is "capable of endless variations" (Jung, 1954/1967, p. 272 [CW13, para. 350]).

Furthermore, these images may not be related to the process of individuation, but to complexes that are not yet dealt with. For Jung, the endless flow of images like the mythic figure of Proteus has to be seized so as it can give its truth. The episode narrated by von Franz about an analysand of Jung's is a good example. She had begun in the following terms:

> I was on a beach by the sea, and a lion was coming toward me. He turned into a ship and was out on the sea [...]. Jung interrupted her. 'Nonsense. When a lion comes toward you, you have a reaction. You don't just wait around and watch until the lion turns into a ship!'
> (Von Franz, 1993, p. 147)

However, some Jungians have challenged the dogma of trying to "pause" the image encountered in oneiric fantasies. The Jungian analyst Rix Weaver described the advantages in not restraining the use of the unfolding of fantasy in active imagination: "sometimes grotesque fantasy that initially lead nowhere can in given time and circumstance, mould into something of real value" (Weaver, 1973, pp. 16–17). The psyche does not just tell a story here and an entirely unrelated episode there. Although the fantasy parts seem unrelated, there is a thread that ties them together. Therefore, for some Jungians, "grotesque fantasy" like RED's imaginative fabulations can also have their place in helping the patient individuate. Given Jung's need to move away from Freud and his free-associative method, Jungians have been wary of allowing freer movement of images on the imaginative plane. On the contrary, in RED, the presence of the analyst allows the patient to let things happen more in the oneiric space since the therapist will know if the patient is moving too fast without making good contact with the environs as he describes what he is seeing *a vive voce*.

Implications of imaginative movement for a RED-based active imagination

In contrast to Desoille, the Jungian therapist or analyst would find it more difficult to be directive since he or she would avoid to point the patient towards any particular direction to be taken. Jung stated that if the therapist forces "the analysis [...] to follow a systematic course, it is a gross mistake in technique" (Jung, 1914/1961 p. 272 [*CW*4, para. 625]).). If anything, Jungians tend to give more importance to the depths than to heights. Furthermore, the Swiss Jungian analyst Tina Keller (1941), who was familiar with both active imagination and *rêve éveillé dirigé,* warns against the use of heights for "*intellcuals*/intellectuals" and recommends "*de descendre pur se rapprocher de la realite'concrete*/to go down to approach reality" (Keller, 1941, p. 81).

I think it is clinically very interesting that images tend to morph when moved upwards; however, from an analytical psychological perspective, we have to avoid quickly trying to alter the negative images into positive ones. Sometimes the therapist has to encourage the subject to do what he or she at first does not want to do, such as address the menacing figures, jump into the darkness and speak to strangers. While, as practitioners, it is good to know the dynamics of oneiric space (and to this we are also grateful to Desoille who manages to give a detailed exposition of the "height trips"), we must also resist our premature impulse to bring the patient to a comfortable, safe ending. We also have to hold our curiosity in seeing what inanimate figures and animals represent in the real life of the patient. As Jungians we have to stay with the unfathomable analogical richness of the image and avoid a reductionistic approach to discover the meanings of images.

The main focus in our framework, when it comes to exploring imaginative oneiric space, should be on a general stimulation for the patient to explore the imaginative landscape with all his or her senses. RED has the benefit of adding a running commentary to the imaginative activity taking place in front of the patient's inner eyes. A RED-based active imagination will be characterised by both movement and resting in the oneiric space than by inner dialogues with encountered figures in the oneiric landscape, as is the case with classic active imagination. Yet, the therapist's presence can ensure that even in the most imaginative flights, there is always a holding back that guarantees a more engaging imaginative experience. Furthermore, in a RED-based active imagination, the therapist should aim to maintain the right tension between holding and moving the image, given the diverse nature of patients' character styles. Some patients cannot move away from fixed images, while others easily produce oneiric dramas.

At the same time, it is worth noting that from a Jungian perspective, action for the sake of action is not crucial. The main focus should remain on the emotions experienced during the waking dream, which in themselves move us psychically. An honest encounter and engagement with the symbols by approaching, perceiving, experiencing and looking at them should remain the characteristic of our theoretical framework. Here, Jung's caveat is very relevant. In the *Visions Seminars*, he states: "So in these visions you may get the surface, but the essence is not necessarily experienced" (Jung, 1998, p. 919). Jung also states that what is most important is not "the object of a vision but the way in which one has perceived the thing" (ibid., p. 920).

Imaginative holding

The ideas of support and safety offered by the therapist are associated with Winnicott's (1960) concept of "holding" and Bion's (1962) idea of containment. Just as a parent attunes to the needs of a baby, so the therapist can provide the patient with necessary support to do the work of psychotherapy. This kind of therapeutic support also applies to when the patient is engaged in an imaginative experience. I refer to this form of support as "imaginative holding." We will now be seeing to what extent and in what form this is offered in RED and active imagination.

Imaginative holding in RED

Desoille's RED seems to be very supportive of the patient to face one's dark side, and Desoille claimed that he had cured patients who had failed to recover with psychoanalysis. In RED, the patient undertakes a gradual regression, emboldened by the therapist's sense of security. As a holding environment, RED can serve as reparative space for psychological trauma. At times, when the scenario becomes too threatening for the patient, the patient will try to find a way out, so as not to face the menacing images. Desoille would offer the patients protective objects of *"caractère magique/* magical character" to face the fearful situation, or encourage the patients to ask the menacing figures who they were, or what they wanted from them. Alternatively, Desoille would also ask the patients to imagine him beside them. These anxiety-reducing techniques[7] of Desoille's RED today resemble Wolpe's use of desensitisation, especially in the forms developed by Lazarus, such as using "emotive imagery." Desoille (1955) believed that one had to speak to the imaginary by using its own language. Desoille follows Janet's early hypno-therapeutic attempts with hysterics, in which he would enter into his patient's imagery and help them by changing the basic pathological structure of the fantasy experience.

Other post-Desoillians (Virel & Fretigny, 1968; Balzarini, 1985) ask the patients to physically ground their imaginative self by becoming more aware of their imaginative surrogate ego, especially the feet, so as to be more grounded. Virel and Fretigny (1968) would encourage the patient to move out of the immersive imaginative experience by just watching it as if watching a film. This distancing technique has been recently utilised when trauma patients are flooded with visual flash backs of traumatic content (Reddemann, 2008). The "screen technique" and the "observer technique" are examples of such distancing methods. Kluft (1989) also describes several "temporizing techniques," including imaginative ones, so as to offer the patient respite and temporary asylum needed to regain mastery and self-efficacy. In fact, given Jung's caveat of losing oneself in the unconscious, all therapists should be very careful as to how to allow patients to explore their darkest sides. Desoille's RED and the developments of his disciples seem to offer examples of how to take such risks in therapy.

Imaginative holding in active imagination

Jung stated that in facing the unconscious difficulties one has to "renounce one's will [...] and do nothing but wait and trust to the impersonal power of growth and development" (Jung, 1998, p. 321). For Jung in therapy: "There are no magical cures for neurosis" (Jung, 1916/1966, p. 293 [CW7, para. 497]). The only magic is in the numinous image itself which plays magician in the sense of conjoining disparate parts of ourselves, consciousness and unconsciousness. Jung's words seem to echo those of St. Theresa of Avila in her *Interior Castle*: "In sum, there is no remedy in this tempest, but to wait for the mercy of God [...]" (Avila, 1979, p. 113). In fact, there is an aspect of creative expression that can only be born through great suffering. When we engage in expressing that suffering in any way shape or form, we are aligning ourselves with the archetype of the wounded healer.

In facing one's own issues, one has to overcome the temptation of finding quick fixes, as Von Franz accuses Desoille, Leuner and Happich amongst others of doing in their directed waking dream methodologies (von Franz, 1980). In *The Red Book*, Jung insisted that living one's own life is a difficult task, as the "the way leads through the crucified" (Jung, 2009, p. 310). For Jung, if one is to carry out a personal transformation, he or she has to let oneself experience that which is scary, if need be, to be bitten by wild animals without running away from them. In doing this, one would be exposing oneself to the instinctual impulses of the unconscious without identifying with them or having them flee back to the unconscious (Dieckmann, 1997). The ordeals and trials that we face in our life and which we can experience in our waking dreams put us "through the fire," initiating

us into undeveloped higher transpersonal potentials. Whether the fire puri-
fies or destroys us depends upon our inner resources and capacities.

Implications of imaginative holding in a RED-based active imagination

Desoille's element of directivity caused a lot of polemics during his time and
after his death, and is probably the main aspect which Jungians resist. However, I believe that Jung's choice of the word "active" in active imagination
should allow more room for the ego to participate actively within the imaginative scenarios, since the ego plays a crucial part in the transformation
of consciousness with its interaction with unconscious material. Furthermore, the therapist can be facilitative rather than directive by employing
"socratic imagery" (in contrast to guided imagery). Socratic imagery is the
imagery version of Socratic questioning applied in the context of imagery
modification whereby patients are encouraged to create their own mastery/
coping imagery, as well as their own self-calming/self-nurturing imagery
(Smucker, 1997). Such a technique gives responsibility to the patient to get
in touch with his or her own inner physician. On a similar note, Edith
Kramer speaks of the "third hand" in art therapy, which supports "the
creative process along without being intrusive, without distorting meaning or imposing pictorial ideas or preferences alien to the client" (Kramer,
2000, p. 48). Post-Desoillians ask the patients themselves to look for objects which might be helpful, rather than suggesting them directly. This is
similar to Jung's ideas when he made reference to stories of heroes who find
themselves in predicaments. Suddenly an animal would appear and lead the
hero to safety. Things very near and evident are often overlooked, such as
instincts, which are often represented by animals. Such resources appear
with a logic of their own.

Fairy tales themselves, which are studied by Jungians, can also be used
for ideas when patients are faced with threatening figures. The duality and
co-existence of constructive and destructive inner energies of the human
psyche are so well expressed in fairy tales. Von Franz's (1974) work on fairy
tales clearly shows how the personal and collective shadow is represented in
fairy tale symbols. Very often in fairy tales, the repressed aspects of one's
soul, wants to be seen and recognised in order to dissolve, or become less
dangerous. The thorough Jungian knowledge of fairy tales can better equip
the therapist to deal with sinister figures rather than the quick move to clear
danger with, for example, a magic wand, as we sometimes find in RED.
Fairy tales themselves indicate that the hero on a quest has to go through
a lot of challenges before he manages to achieve his mission. At the same
time, it is also true that inner helpers and guides, in human or animal form,
can sometimes guide the patients more directly and skilfully on their imagery journey than the therapist is able to do from the outside. These inner

guides can be seen as personifications of the patients' own unconscious inner wisdom and potential. The fantastical dramas of waking dreams can allow Jungians to integrate their knowledge of fairy tales and use them in another innovative way besides their use in amplification or in Dieckmann's (1986) method of exposing adult neurosis via their favourite fairy tale.

These two different approaches of dealing with the unconscious, either by offering support or by leaving the patient to his or her own devices in waking dreams, are archetypally represented by the figures of Merlin/ Trickster and Christ. Merlin is the technical virtuoso. He has an uncanny habit of making challenging problems disappear with a turn of a phrase and a waving of his magic wand. When Merlin brings about change or healing, he confirms his occult powers. Christ, however, is not deemed a magician by Catholics, although Smith (1978) in his book *Jesus the Magician* has argued against this. According to Mogenson (1992), Jesus could have saved himself from the cross since he was also a God, but he endured the suffering of crucifixion. Christ's goal, in contrast to Merlin, was not to exalt himself as a power above all others, but to empower others to live their lives more fully However, it is important to remember that if Jungians distance themselves formally from their own manipulative power, there is the danger that we may unconsciously enact these very qualities even while we naively think ourselves to be on the side of "Christ," i.e., the good ones. For Jung, the "paradoxical nature of Mercurius reflects an important aspect of the Self" and he further notes that the trickster is "a forerunner of the saviour" (Jung, 1954/1968, p. 263 [CW9, para. 472]).

Notes

1 The term refers to the imagined embodied perceptual representations of oneself when engaging in a waking dream.
2 RED can fit in both the discharge model and the process model described in Totton's (2003) *Body Psychotherapy: An Introduction*. The discharge model describes how the body therapy can be used for emotional expression while the process model aims to sensitively facilitate the healing and psychological growth process latent in the body.
3 Swami Siddheswarananda (1897–1957) was a respected monk of the Ramakrishna Mission or Vedanta Mission. He was the representative of the French Vedantic school created by Vivekananda and continued by Auribondo Ghose (Choisy, 1949).
4 Enargeic comes from the Greek rhetorical term *enargeia* which refers to a visually powerful description that vividly recreates something or someone in words.
5 Modern Devotion was a movement for religious reform, calling for apostolic renewal through the rediscovery of genuine pious practices such as humility, obedience and simplicity of life. It began in the late fourteenth century, largely through the work of Gerard Groote, and flourished in the Low Countries and Germany in the fifteenth century, but came to an end with the Protestant Reformation. It is most known today through its influence on Thomas à Kempis,

the author of *The Imitation of Christ*, a book which proved highly influential for centuries. For further information, see J.H. Van Engen's (1988) *Devotio Moderna*.

6 Milton Erickson (1901–1980) was an American psychiatrist who specialised in medical hypnosis and family therapy. He was the founding president of the American Society for Clinical Hypnosis and noted for his approach to the unconscious mind as creative and solution-generating. Erickson believed that the unconscious mind was always listening, and that, whether or not the patient was in trance, suggestions could be made which would have a hypnotic influence, as long as those suggestions found some resonance at the unconscious level. The Ericksonian approach departs from traditional hypnosis in a variety of ways. While the process of hypnosis has customarily been conceptualised as a matter of the therapist issuing standardised instructions to a passive patient, Ericksonian hypnosis stresses the importance of the interactive therapeutic relationship and purposeful engagement of the inner resources and experiential life of the subject. For further information, see Jay Haley's (1993) book *Milton H. Erickson. A Brief Biography*.

7 Direct intervention into the waking dream itself is similar to Neo-Senoi techniques, which manipulate or destroy threatening dreams or mental images. Currently, there is a growing literature on the amelioration and healing of pathological conditions by such deliberately manipulative methods (Larsen, 1996). For example in the "Simonton method" (Simmonton, Matthews-Simmonton & Creighton, 1978) which is used in palliative care, the patient is encouraged to imagine that he or she is fighting a battle between invasive or cancerous forces and the body's defences. In the imagery, the patient is encouraged to win over the defences by eating or driving away the negative forces.

Chapter 14

A theoretical comparison of RED and active imagination

Transferential issues, narrative style and interpretation in the middle and final phase of treatment

Three other concepts namely transferential and counter-transferential relationship, narratives and interpretation will help to complete the comparison aimed to elicit the commonalities and divergences between RED and active imagination. These categories are more related to the middle and final phase of treatment.

Solitude a deux: the interplay of transference and counter-transference

Traditionally, transference and counter-transference are located distinctly in the psychoanalytic tradition. The original concept of transference stems from hypnosis and an understanding of the power of suggestion (Ellenberger, 1970). While Freud wrote extensively about transference as a redirection of feelings about some significant person from the past on to the analyst, he wrote very little on the phenomenon of counter-transference. In *Analysis Terminable and Interminable*, Freud (1937/1950) identified it as an experience existing within the analyst and as a limiting factor in analytic work. This contrasted with Jung's view of psychotherapy as a two-way interaction in which the patient and the therapist are both deeply emotionally involved in and affected by the therapeutic situation, which was quite radical in Jung's time (Samuels, 1985, 2008). Jung emphasised the critical healing value of unconscious communication between patient and therapist, a phenomenon otherwise known as the transference-counter-transference dynamic (Samuels, 2006; Perry, 2008). More specifically, Jung was important in recognising the potential clinical utility of counter-transference, describing it as a "highly important organ of information" (Jung, 1931/1966, p. 71 [CW16, para. 163]) to be used by therapists.

Today, many relational and intersubjective psychoanalytic models embrace the notion of mutual influence and acknowledge the unavoidable involvement of the analyst's subjectivity in the therapeutic process (Mitchell, 1988, 2000; Gill, 1994; Aron, 1996; Hoffman, 1998; Bromberg, 2001; Safran & Muran, 2002; Wachtel, 2008; Safran, 2012; Ferro & Civitarese, 2015). In the contemporary psychoanalytic view, counter-transference is seen as an occurrence that happens because of both the therapist's and patient's contributions. The therapist brings his or her own history into the relationship but the patient can also induce feelings within the therapist (Gabbard, 2004).

Post-Jungians have also developed ideas about counter-transference over the years, many of which complement contributions to counter-transference theory made by notable psychoanalysts such as Robert Langs, Margaret Little, Paula Heimann, Heinrich Racker and Harold Searles (for reviews see Sedgwick, 1994; Machtiger, 1995; Samuels, 2006; Perry, 2008; Wiener, 2009). Furthermore, many contemporary Jungians, particularly those influenced by developmental and psychodynamic theory, increasingly focus on the transference-counter-transference field as the primary site of therapeutic action in their clinical work (Sedgwick, 2001; Samuels, 2008; Solomon, 2008). I will now describe the role that transference and counter-transference dynamics play in RED and active imagination.

The therapeutic relationship in RED

In RED the use of transference and counter-transference in the therapeutic relationship was rather restricted since Desoille's method offered an alternative to psychoanalysis which based its method of treatment on the transference dynamics. For Desoille, the transference itself is played out in the images that come up during the oneiric drama that the patient engages in: *"Dans le rêve éveillé dirigé, le transfert se passe avant tout dans le rêve éveillé lui-même*/In the directed waking dream, the transference passes through the waking dream itself" (Desoille et al., 1966, p. 66). The Argentinian post-Desoillian Rocca (1984) also developed *"el circuito de la directividad*/the circuit of directivity," a two-way circular therapeutic relationship between patient and analyst which moves beyond the linear model of therapist-patient interaction but still lacks the depth of the Jungian interactive therapeutic relationship.

Later on, after Desoille's death, post-Desoillians, especially in the psychoanalytic group G.I.R.E.P., explored the *rêve éveillé* itself as a third pole besides the pole of the analyst and the other pole of the patient. The idea of the third pole was linked to the classic Oedipal constellation (Freud, 1905; Klein, 1928; Britton, 1989). The waking dream enables the fostering of the third position of the Oedipal triangle, in that it creates a triangular interaction (Launey, Levine & Maurey, 1975). Additional conceptualisations by the G.I.R.E.P. group include the Winnicottian triangle of mother, child and transitional object (1958/1971), superimposed onto the waking dream-patient-analyst triangle (Fabre, 1979; Fabre & Maurey, 1985). These ideas of G.I.R.E.P. pre-empted to a certain extent the concept of triangular relationship in art therapy (Wood, 1984, 1990; Dalley, Rifkind & Terry, 1993; Schaverien, 2000; Case, 2000). The G.I.R.E.P. group was heavily influenced by the so-called "British independent school" in psychoanalysis

(Fabre, 1979, 1982), especially with ideas of "holding environment," "transitional object" and "pre-oedipal conflicts" which they applied to their waking dream method. The analyst is often described as a mother who is "playing" with the patient-child who is offered the waking dream. The waking dream was seen as a way of becoming aware of the deficits and impingement in the pre-oedipal phase of the parent-child relationship. Moreover, the experience of sharing the waking dream directly with the therapist provides a way for the patient to integrate such emotional deficits. The "good-enough" therapist holds the child-patient by attuning and supporting the patient in the waking dream. The waking dream itself offers the patient a potential space to recreate a sense of illusion, which is important to have as a child, but because of parental impingement this could not be developed. The therapist allows the patient to hold the illusion but tries to transition him or her to a sense of reality through the frame of the session, without creating too much frustration.

Active imagination, transference and counter-transference

In analytical psychology, complexes do not just appear as symbols but also manifest in relationships, including the therapeutic relationship with its transferences and counter-transferences. Late in his career, Jung (1916/1957) relaxed his view that active imagination has to be practised alone and stated that it "[...] could just as well take place between patient and analyst" (CW 8, para. 186, p. 89). However, he did not amplify more on the subject and it was up to the post-Jungians (Champernowne, 1969; Whitehouse, 1979; Kalf, 1980; Schaverien, 1982, 1991, 2005; Woodman, 1982; Chodorow, 1995; Edwards, 2010) to open this idea in the Jungian creative arts. In fact, the latter built upon Jung's ideas of the transference and counter-transference dynamics of the analytic setting.

It is in the alchemical text, *Rosarium Philosophorum*,[1] that Jung found a symbolic representation of this dialectic between the unconscious of the analyst and that of the patient. In the analytic situation, there is a deep connection of the analyst's unconscious with the client's unconscious and this is, according to Jungian theory, a necessary condition for transformative healing to occur (Sedgwick, 1994). The unconscious-to-unconscious bond is characterised by powerful, shifting transference-counter-transference dynamics and thus brings to the forefront the notion of the analyst-as-wounded healer. The analyst in this situation tries to work on the patient by working on him- or herself, continuously addressing his or her own difficulties, or counter-transference, in relation to the patient (Sedgwick, 1994, 2001). As Jung (1931/1966) stated, "the doctor must change himself if he is to become capable of changing his patient" (Jung, 1931/1966, p. 73 [CW16, para. 170]).

Wiener describes how analysts must create a "shared mental space" (Weiner, 2009, pp. 69–74) in the imagination where something new and meaningful is allowed to emerge, a concept similar to Ogden's (1994) "analytic third" and the lesser-known "subtle body" (Schwartz-Salant, 1986) or "interactive field" in Jungian contexts (Schwartz-Salant, 1988, 1989, 1995). These imaginative uses of counter-transference require the analyst to make all of him- or herself available to the unconscious, using feelings, thoughts, bodily responses, images and dreams to understand the patient (Davidson, 1966; Schaverien, 2005, 2007, 2008; Wiener, 2009). Schaverien (2007, 2008) proposes that when images, fantasies or bodily sensations arise in the counter-transference that seems to have no obvious or easily identifiable source or meaning, analysts may benefit from using imaginative processes to discover what these may be trying to communicate. Schaverien (2007, 2008) views this process as doing the traditional Jungian active imagination. By staying imaginatively open to the unconscious, something entirely new sometimes emerges in the transference-counter-transference dynamic, what Jung would describe as the transcendent function (Davidson, 1966; Sedgwick, 1994, 2001; Carter, 2010; Schaverien, 2007). This new or third factor may help facilitate change from one psychological attitude to another, healthier one (Sedgwick, 1994, 2001; Schaverien, 2007, 2008). This psychological change tends to manifest as the patient and therapist experience a more open communication with the unconscious, and an increased capacity to symbolise and tolerate ambiguity, all signs of progress in individuation (Davidson, 1966; Sedgwick, 1994, 2001; Stein, 2006; Schaverien, 2007, 2008).

Schaverien introduces art to the intermediary area between therapist and patient and how this affects transference and counter-transference. She writes:

> The pictures may be an additional catalyst for such an unconscious meeting because they too hold projections and are the channel through which the activated unconscious may be diverted. [...] Thus, the combination of client–picture-therapist may be a highly charged triangular encounter. It may be that intense transference projections are deflected into the picture. In some cases this will mean there is a less intense transference to the person of the therapist.
>
> (Schaverien, 1999, pp. 119–120)

Schaverien describes that the picture may reveal the inner emotional landscape of the patient but she also adds: "The picture mediates in the therapeutic relationship and has considerable influence on it" (ibid., p. 117). Moreover, Schaverien also speaks of "aesthetic counter-transference," that is, the effects the picture has on the art therapist/viewer, as well as the client. She emphasises that the picture may exhibit the transference "but it can only evoke counter-transference" (ibid., p. 121). In analytical art therapy, the entire space within the triangular therapeutic, i.e., client-therapist image, becomes a kind of three-dimensional field of transference-counter-transference exchange. Here, active within the therapeutic space are the client transference to the therapist as well as to the art (Schaverien, 1987, 1999), the therapist's unconscious reactions to the client (counter-transference) and the phenomenon of "aesthetic counter-transference" both from the client and the therapist towards the art, creating a full therapeutic triangular dynamic (Schaverien, 2000). Other writers have explored the particular dynamics of transference, counter-transference and aesthetic counter-transference within the triangular relationship in art therapy (Wood, 1990; Simon, 1995; Case, 2000; Schaverien, 2000).

One of the few analysts who write about active imagination in the an-alytic setting, Anne Marie Kroke (2004), is influenced by "Guided Affec-tive Imagery" of Hanscarl Leuner. Kroke describes how she makes use of her counter-transference by listening to any sensations and images that she has in the moment before the patient enters the waking dream. In another article (2013), she describes how she silently witnesses the unfolding of the waking dream until she perceives that interrupted dialogue and the defences that interrupt the flow of the imaginative content. Kroke takes note of what is *"evitato, adombrato, scisso o altro*/avoided, hidden, split or other" (ibid., p. 76) and decides whether to leave it for another time or else to present it as a stimulus to the patient so as to be able to overcome the defences. While post-Jungians have written extensively on the transference and counter-transference dynamics in the analytic setting, very little has been applied to the visualisation modality of active imagination in session in contrast to other forms of Jungian creative arts.

Implications of transference and counter-transference in a RED-based active imagination

I feel that the Jungian conception of an interactive field can be very helpful in deepening the formulation of an active visual imagination in the analytic setting. At face value, in a waking dream, the patient "dreams" in order to "awaken" while "alone" in the presence of the therapist (Winnicott, 1958). One can describe this solitude as a form of relational solitude as a *solitude a deux*. However, the therapist, patient and waking dream are not separate, but are indivisible and interactive parts of a greater unified field. In fact, the waking dream of the patient can be considered a waking dream within a big-ger waking dream emanating from the therapeutic field. In practising active imagination in the analytic setting, the waking dream is also considered as forming a triangular relationship between the patient and the therapist and which can embody transference reactions to the therapist. Furthermore, it can also lead to direct transference and counter-transference both by the therapist and the patient, who may react to it when he or she sits with it at a later stage, especially if he or she puts it in writing or art form, or avoids engaging with it. The counter-transferential dynamics are similar to those explained by Schaverien in analytic art therapy that is "aesthetic counter-transference," but instead of emanating from the picture, it is elicited from the waking dream.

The waking dream in the analytic setting can lead to a counter-transference from the therapist who is actively listening and has time to absorb the unfolding of the waking dream. Sedgwick describes how the analyst must "clear the field" (Sedgwick, 1994, p. 122) so as to attune to whatever emerges from the patient's and their own unconscious. Sedgwick (1994) referred to this process as incubating while Milner (1950) refers to it as a "wide-unfocused state." The therapist can use the steps of Schaverien (2007) to make sense of the images, sensations and thoughts experienced in counter-transference. The ability to recognise this becomes key to the therapist of how to become active, lucid or directive in the waking dream experienced in the therapy room.

In fact, from the post-Desoillians, we can take it a step further by using the counter-transference and give it back to the patient in the form of a stimulus. When both parties involved in the transference recognise this, they can collaboratively transform and deepen the shared waking dream they are having. Therefore, the patient also has his or her own turn giving a "stimulus" to the therapist to reverie upon through the therapeutic field, which then allows the unconscious to resume its revelatory function. Kroke's (2013) input on feeding back to the patient the moment when he or she interrupts the waking dream can also be useful.

Therapist and patient are dreaming up the field, while at the same time in a circular rather than a linear process, the field is dreaming them up. Something deeper is revealing itself through their interplay and sharing of conscious and unconscious material. What is moving in the imagination of the patient while dreaming awake touches something in the therapist, such as his or her thoughts, sensations, fantasies and dreams. Jung spoke of "psychic infection" (Jung, 1937/1966, p. 329 [CW16, para. 545]). The imagination springs forth between the patient and the therapist. Dreaming their shared process in the interactive field becomes a truly embodied alchemical "coniunctio," a coming together of the opposites, an incarnation of the Self, in real time and space. While the idea of giving back a stimulus to the patient from one's own counter-transference and to ask him or her to start another waking dream comes from the post-Desoillians, the idea of circularity in the interactive field of post-Jungians definitely enriches the post-Desoillian understanding of how to make better use of the analytic setting.

Narratives

The concept of narrative in therapy can be divided between: psychodynamic and cognitive/constructivist approaches, and constructionist ones.

The first one employs narrative and story as a means of gaining access to personality structures. For example, a client-centred therapist will listen to a story for evidence of self-acceptance while a psychodynamic one will listen for data that inform patterns of conflict (Strupp & Binder, 1984; Luborsky & Crits-Christoph, 1990), object relations and attachment styles (Holmes, 1993). The second approach emphasises the role of narrative and story-telling in lives and relationships. Thus, narrative is put at the heart of therapy where narrative becomes therapy itself (White & Epston, 1990). Both approaches are interested in meaning-making, but while the first approach locates meaning within a foundational structure of the person, the constructionists view meaning as a social construction and a relational activity (McNamee & Gergen, 1999; McNamee, 2002). The latter directs our attention to language practices as opposed to private thoughts. Neimeyer (2000) identifies the constructivist narrative as intrapersonally focused, while constructionist narrative is interpersonally focused. Constructionists describe narratives as forms of action, as social performances. They are not, as more cognitively oriented constructivists would claim, causal schemas explaining our actions.

RED and narratives

In Desoillian RED, narrative is a main part of the method and patients open up more easily to their therapist given RED's dis-inhibitive effect. RED uses extended visual fantasies in narrative form to obtain information about the motivational system of the individual, including elements of conflict, perceptual distortion, self-perception and early memories. RED seems to use the narrative *in vivo* itself as a form of "enactment" that becomes part of the imaginative activity, leaving no real separation between the intrapsychic drama and the external enactment. Thus, RED offers both a narrative which can be perused for evaluating the patient's personality, and narrative as a performance between therapist and patient, opening it to the relational. The patient's private reverie transforms into a public statement through his or her *ekphrasis* of the oneirodrama. Desoille kept a good balance between the visual and the verbal, transcending both Freud's iconoclasm and Lacan's emphasis on linguistic structuralism. Fabre and Maurey mention the narrative component "*le verbe*" when she described the Desoillian waking dream as made up of three Vs: "*le vivre, le voir et le verbe*/to experience, to see and to verbalise" (Fabre & Maurey, 1985, p. 223). In RED, the therapist encourages the patient to talk and pose questions to encountered images in internal space. The patient does this in a way that is heard by the therapist. The patient in RED acts somewhat like a medium in a séance as Jung has very well described in the early studies of his career on his cousin Helen Preiswerk, who would channel the messages heard and passed by spirits to the séance group members. The narrative itself helps provide a form of containment for the patient, a protection against the dissolving influence of the subjective inner world, and helps the analyst keep track of the patient's inner journey and to formulate a proper diagnosis. In RED, besides the therapist's recording of the waking dreams, the patients are encouraged to write down their own narrative of their waking dream, their personal myth, once they go home, and to record the dreams between sessions, thus keeping a balanced tension between images and words. RED therapy seeks to employ the voice besides images as a primary channel through which to lure exiled images and dissociated aspects of the psyche into consciousness. Several art therapists (Baron, 1989; Lusebrink, 1990; Jones, Vinton & Wernick, 1999) have used guided imagery as a means to facilitate art engagement. Usually after being asked to imagine, the patient is asked to draw what he or she has visualised. In the directed waking dream, the visualisation is not drawn (although it can be drawn at a later stage), but voiced simultaneously. In RED, external images can also be used as visual "prompts" to start an imaginative experience. While art therapists argue that the external creation is better than just visualisation (Lusebrink, 1990; Schaverien, 1999) since it adds a two- or three-dimensional representation of the image, the directed waking dream relies instead on the use of both visualisation and the spoken narrative, in the presence of the therapist. Ironically, art therapists also use the externalised painted image to speak about it or to open a conversation on certain issues portrayed. The directed waking dream builds on the idea that persons think both in words and in images.

Edward Sapir (1921) pointed to the differences between voice and speech, proposing that speech is about the subject matter and choice of vocabulary, while voice relates to the way in which this is uttered. A person's flow of words provides precise information about the flow of life in all aspects of his or her existence. Sometimes too much verbosity and verbal agility in the waking dream try to seduce the inner journey one is called to do. The qualities of the patient's voice need to be perceived in terms of their synaesthetic imagery, i.e., their taste, their colour, their sound, their smell or touch so as to be represented more fully. Raised and lowered tones, sudden silence, hesitancies and changes in volume must be individually examined to reveal defiance and resistance. The Argentian post-Desoillian Andres Cafferata[2] has come up with a classification of how attention to the choice of language and process of narration can give important clues to the analyst about the inner world of the patient. Cafferata describes different styles of the patient's narration which are characteristic of the obsessive, hysteric, narcissistic and psychosomatic patient (Rocca & Villamarin, 2008). The words and the tonalities in which we express our words are based on a broad range of functioning such as our brain and neurological functioning which reveal our emotional states, our intellectual use of cognitive processes and the cultural realm in which we live. The voice is always in attendance and tells us who we are. Furthermore, the voice, as the speaker of our identity, becomes an aural mirror and expression of our soul since it allows repressed images in the soul to be spoken and heard.

Active imagination and narratives

The narrative aspect of Jungian analysis has not been as thoroughly critiqued as Roy Schafer (1980) has done for psychoanalysis. Some Jungian scholars have found a confluence between his thought and "narrative" ideas (Pietikaninen, 1999) or postmodernism[3] (Hauke, 2000). Yet the connections are not so obvious from the other side. One of the features of Jungian analysis is its view of narrative as being primarily internal, made up of an internal landscape of one's dreams, fantasies and other archetypal experiences. We are called to understand ourselves through the images our psyches create and the narrative fictions that follow from them (Hillman, 1983). Usually, the content of this imaginative material is made up of quests, journeys and self-transformation. The plot is forward-looking and full of several mythic themes that never fit one particular model story, such as the Oedipus myth.

For Jung, the psyche is a spontaneous storyteller. Jung stated in the *Visions Seminars*, "The soul is always supposed to come from the mouth, the spirit comes out of words" (Jung, 1998, p. 251). The image is trusted to lead the way to a healing narrative, rather than towards the ego's wish to cover, explain and analyse. Active imagination is a way of tapping into this drama. It is like a series of scenes from a mystery, or acts from an ongoing play with no set script. The person experiencing the fantasy improvises as he or she changes with the spontaneous development of the plot. Jung (2009) gave us his own experience of the fantasies he engaged with in *The Red Book*.

Jung's (2009) *The Red Book* is full of dialogues with personified unconscious images which form separate narratives in the three chapters. Jung engaged in several dialogues with these unconscious figures such as with Izdubar and Philemon. Jung believed that in personifying unconscious figures, one could really confront the unconscious. Jung, like Desoille, also believed that it was important to write down one's fantasies. However, Jung (1963/1995) went for "high flown language" so as to be better able to understand them.

Implications of narrative in a RED-based active imagination

Through RED, Jungians can employ the use of the therapist as an aural mirror and acoustic echo of the patient's inner journey. Through the patient's ekphrastic narrative, the patient fulfils a need to tell his or her personal myth in front of an "other," incarnating Schelling's metaphor that "language itself is a mythology" (Bachelard, 1960, p. 37). Furthermore, the description of the waking dream helps to create a sense of "community," bridging the gap that separates the patient from the therapist.

Another value of vivid, detailed description of the waking dream lies in prompting linear left brain thinking while employing nonlinear right brain thinking at the same time. This helps to achieve a balance and an integration of these two activities, for example, in the case of unprocessed traumatic episodes. Trauma is associated with disruptions in imagery and memory and traumatic memories are often stored as imagery and body sensation (Gantt & Tinnin, 2009), making expressive therapies compatible to work with these aspects of trauma (Appleton, 2011). When words cannot integrate the disorganised sensations and action patterns that form the core imprint of the trauma (van der Kolk, 2014), the waking dream helps the patient to start verbalising after first accessing certain sensations and images connected to the trauma (Valtorta and Passerini, 2015). What Rossi (1990) said about fine literature and poetry, namely that they are a form by which the words of the left hemisphere give voice to the symbols and archetypal patterns of the right, can be equally valid for the directed waking dream.

The therapist can benefit in learning to receive and work with images in the patient's voice, and with voice as image itself. Analytic-oriented music therapists such as Paul Newham (1993), Noah Pikes (2005), as well as Diane Austin (2006) have also developed voice work as a form of active imagination, building on the work of Alfred Wolfsohn. This possibility is also offered in RED. The ekphrastic narrative is not only expressive but also creative, involving the listener on many levels. It is a form of entrancement, an *ekstasis* leading to a moment of sublime rupture in the listening therapist. In the Middle Ages, the most refined sense that established the best contact with the world was hearing, sight came in only third place after touch before it became the prime organ of perception in the last centuries. In the sixteenth century the church based its authority on the word, faith is hearing: *"auditum verbi Dei, id est fidem*, the ear, the ear alone, Luther said is the Christian organ" (Barthes, 1989, p. 67). It is precisely the intersubjectivity that these narratives perform that make the somatic aspects of language worthy of attention. The ekphrastic narrative of the waking dream can actively captivate the listening therapist and turn the waking dream into a visual and vocal rhetoric.

Besides asking the patient to write down his or her waking fantasy, the therapist can ask the patient to draw the visual narrative, replete with different scenes and figures. When carrying out active imagination, several Jungians (Dallett, 1982, 2008; Johnson, 1986, and Raff, 2006) believe it is important to draw the images as well as writing the dialogues one has had in his or her fantasy experience. Such a procedure could ensure that the patient can continue to capture and engage his or her oneiric fantasies.

Interpretation

Interpretation is usually associated with Freudian psychoanalysis. It was considered the main intervention of the analyst and the driving force of therapeutic change. Freud linked change to the insight obtained through interpretation, seen as the clarification of a hidden meaning. However, classical interpretation today appears less important for the purposes of change than was traditionally thought. Some have even underlined the negative impact of interpretation, for instance, with borderline and psychotic patients (Rosenfeld, 1987; McWilliams, 1994). The trend in therapy is one of showing more caution in interpreting than was previously recommended. We will now describe and discuss Desoille and Jung's views on interpretation.

RED and interpretation

The primary assumption in RED is that the symbolism inherent in visual imagery constitutes an affective "forgotten" language which can express unconscious motives. Although Desoille devoted time to look at these images in a different session, he also believed that insight could happen in the oneiric drama. Desoille believed that a person may be replaced by an object in oneirc space which shows one of his or her own qualities, or else by a symbol similar in emotional value or by a situation analogous to one in which the person had had an important influence upon the psychological development of the individual. According to Desoille, sometimes to arrive at the meaning of a particular image one has to wait for a spontaneous modification or mutation. At times, Desoille would encourage the patient to bring up the object or animal met in the sea depths, where the metamorphosis of the object into a human known person would usually occur. Nonetheless, it is not possible to formulate a reliable lexicon of image substitutions. This was again re-affirmed by the post-Desoillian, Jean Claude Benoit,

> Dans ce monde imaginaire, l'interprétation symbolique est toujours délicate: 'Il n'existe pas de dictionnaire universel des symboles', disait Desoille.
> In this imaginary world, the symbolic interpretation is always delicate: 'There is no universal dictionary of symbols,' Desoille used to say.
> (Benoit, 1973, p. 189)

For Desoille, the oneiric drama itself led to sublimated feelings. The idea that the waking dream itself can become a liberated embodied experience was also expressed by Desoille's disciples, Dr. Marc Guillerey (1954), Favez-Boutonnier (1947), Dr. Jean Claude Benoit (1973), and those groups such as C.I.R.M.E.P. and S.I.T.I.M., who after Desoille's death took his integrated approach into humanistic and somatic psychotherapy. Guillerey wrote that the symbolic expression via his method "est déjà en elle meme liberatrice et curative/is already liberating and curative in itself" (Guillerey, 1955, p. 9). Juliet Favez-Boutonnier, in her thesis titled "L'angoisse/angst," described the cathartic effect of the waking dream as being "indépendant des interpretations/independent of interpretation" given (Favez-Boutonnier,

1947, p. 195). Jean Claude Benoit (1973) also stated that the image itself holds a particular force to co-ordinate, synthesise and regulate the psyche. This view[4] that imagery is in itself transformational was not shared by the Parisian groups G.I.R.E.P., which integrated psychoanalytic ideas in RED, and C.I.P.A., which integrated completely in psychoanalysis. G.I.R.E.P. gives importance to the session where analyst and patient look at the material together and try to find the latent meaning hidden in the images.

Despite the importance given by Desoille to the affective catharsis "*A cote de la valeur plastique des images, il faut condsiderer leur contenu affectif*/Besides the plastic value of images, one has to consider their affective content" (Desoille, 1948, p. 54) and sublimation of the waking dream itself, he still devoted time to go over the imagined scenario. Desoille would ask the patient to write down what he or she had imagined once at home, and to keep track of his or her dreams as well. Then, the patient and the therapist would look again at the waking dream contents in the next session and compare it to his or her daily life difficulties, as well as connecting them to his or her dreams. During this part of the session, the patient and the therapist would sit face to face. Desoille, like Jung, would not interpret the content of the waking dream, but would ask the patient to share what he or she thought about the waking dream's drama since every symbol has a particular meaning to each patient. These ideas of Desoille are not different from Jung's. An interpretation can be placed between the patient and the therapist as the Latin roots of the word indicate (placing/pretere; between/ inter) in a less than conclusive, more poetic way.

The disciple of Desoille, Andre Virel, as well as his colleague, Roger Fretigny (1968), has been firm believers in the diagnostic value of the imaginal responses. They believe that their waking dream procedures allow them to sift out the conflictual material, presenting the individual's fantasy, and to discover the structural details of the individual's personality. However, their method does not yield a typological or nosological report. Fretigny and Virel regard this as an advantage since the technique bypasses typing and connects directly with the ontogenetic roots of the symptomatic feelings and behaviour. Through mental imagery, the difficulty is localised and attached to specific fantasies or events. It can retrace and identify the nature of the emotional trauma, date it and reveal its context. They refer to this as "localisation diagnosis."

Desoille emphasised the importance of finding meaning through symbols in the waking dream together with the patient. However, he also believed that at times insight occurred spontaneously in the waking dream itself as images would morph into human beings from the person's life as they moved upwards along the vertical axis in the waking dream. Desoille also intimated that certain images associated with folklore, mythology or religion would arise from the collective unconscious, as he was influenced by Jung's ideas.

Active imagination and interpretation

Jung understood that symbols, as dream images, do not disguise the meaning of the dream but express exactly what is intended to be the message: "A symbol does not define or explain; it points beyond itself to a meaning that is darkly divined yet still beyond our grasp, and cannot be adequately expressed in the familiar words of our language" (Jung, 1926/1960, p. 336 [CW8, para. 644]). This statement distinguishes Jung from Freud, who believed that dreams are nothing more than our symptomatically disguised desires. Jung's contribution to depth psychology was to look for the wider, deeper meaning of symbols. Jung would say an actual symbol is the best possible description of a relatively unknown but posited thing: "To be effective a symbol must be by its nature unassailable" (Jung, 1921/1971, p. 237 [CW6, para. 401]). Jung (1956) differentiated symbols from signs since: "they are images of contents which for the most part transcend consciousness" (Jung, 1912/1967, p. 77 [CW5, para. 114]). For Jung, a symbol is capable of uniting opposites: "the symbol is the middle way along which the opposites flow together in a new movement, like a watercourse bringing fertility after a long drought" (Jung, 1921/1971, p. 262 [CW6, para. 443]). Symbols are spontaneous products of the archetypal psyche, and have legitimate effects only when they serve to change our psychic state or conscious attitude.

In the *Visions Seminars*, Jung acknowledged the intrinsic power of images since, "If one can at least perceive unconscious contents, that, in itself, is already an asset because it is close to nature and the next step is to admit them" (Jung, 1998, p. 405). Hillman also considers that "each image is its own beginning, its own end, healed by and in itself [...]" (Hillman, 1983, p. 80). Jung argued for the importance of the lived experience of the images since the transcendent can become immanent, not by process of reasoning but through the immediacy of experience: "For the most important thing is not to interpret and understand the fantasies but primarily to experience them" (Jung, 1928/1966, p. 213 [CW7, para. 342]). Moreover, Jung did insist that images "require to be not only rationally integrated with the conscious mind, but morally assimilated" (Jung, 1931/1966, p. 51 [CW16, para. 111]). Kaufman (2009) puts an emphasis on *translating* the image rather than interpreting the image.

But since symbols are polyvalent, it also means that the connotation of a true symbol is not exhausted when we have found some rational formula which will define or explain it. Jung, more than Desoille, seems to have emphasised the need to draw again the imagined experience and to keep on looking at them until some form of meaning is elicited.

Jung's method of amplification of symbolic material is aligned with the natural process of associationism, inviting an exploration around origins, meanings and purpose. Jung (1935/1970) describes amplification as a logical principle, adopting the method of the philologist, i.e., finding parallels in a variety of texts which then establish meaning. When the use of the symbol is combined with verbal creativity, the meaning of the symbol may achieve greater clarification (Gowan, 1975). The symbol invites collaboration between both therapist and patient to find meanings in it. The conjured images in active imagination are not given meaning by the therapist; rather, the therapist works with the practitioner to unpack the emotion, or draw connections between the images and existing archetypes or myths, that may help to provide answers.

Implications of interpretation in a RED-based active imagination

There are many similarities in this category, i.e., how interpretation is used in both RED and active imagination. In RED, there is also a move away from a reductionistic approach of symbols to an anagogic one, which is also the hallmark of analytical psychology. Desoillians, as from a Jungian perspective, also ask for the meaning of the images from the patients themselves. RED practitioners, like Jungians, use amplification of symbolic material to come to a wider understanding of the symbol. Therefore, in a RED-based approach to active imagination, the images can continue to be explored by both therapist and patient in conjunction with associations, discussion and interpretation. The patient's verbal input plays an important part in discovering the meaning of his or her imagery. Affective reactions linked to the imaginative experience have to be weaved in along associated ideas and memories that are then understood in the light of a detailed anamnesis. One aspect which is different, and can be taken up by Jungians from RED, is that while engaged in a waking dream, the aspects of patient's personal complexes in the unconscious can reveal themselves, when figures morph into familiar persons from the life of the patient especially as they move upwards along the vertical axis. RED can help in recognising personal complexes and how they emerge through the patient's particular experience, and how they continue to powerfully influence his or her life.

Another point which RED can lend to active imagination as practised in session with the therapist is by devoting a separate session to the interpretation of the images. This RED procedure blends in well with the tenets of analytical psychology since Jung has encouraged patients to keep on looking at their images in order to understand them better. Therefore, a session dedicated to finding meaning from the images in the waking dream, definitely, has its benefits since it gives time for both patient and therapist to go over the material. It also reduces the tendency of patients to try and seek meaning while engaged in the oneiric drama itself. Given that patients might arrive at insight in the session itself (Salman, 2010), when engaged in the waking dream, they may still want to continue to process it after the oneiric drama is over. This can be done by also bringing in and comparing the patients' nocturnal dreams following their waking dream session. If both therapist and patient compare the written account of the waking dream, they can also see which material might have been omitted and what could have possibly have led this to happen. Interestingly, Susan Rowland, a Jungian scholar who also specialises in literature, has juxtaposed an interpretation of text and close reading as a form of active imagination itself: "Active imagination is a kind of reading when it insists upon symbolic images being treated as the *text of another*" (Rowland, 2013, p. 92). She further sees it as "a practise of magic" (ibid., p. 94), since it encourages the image to reveal its potential being in the soul spontaneously. Thus, the reviewing of the waking dream written text in the next session can also be seen as an extension of the practice of active imagination.

Another useful aspect of RED which can be integrated with the active imagination conducted in session is the knowledge of how resistance can manifest in imagery, for example through weak images, and incomplete figures, to mention a couple. This Desoillian knowledge can help Jungians to give meaning to these images when they are looked at collaboratively after the session.

Notes

1 *The Rosary of the Philosophers (Rosarium philosophorum sive pretiosissimum donum Dei)* is a sixteenth-century alchemical treatise. It was published in 1550 as Part II of *De Alchimia Opuscula complura veterum philosophorum* (Frankfurt). The term *rosary* in the title refers to a "rose garden," metaphoric of an anthology or collection of wise sayings. The 1550 print includes a series of 20 woodcuts with German-language captions, plus a title page showing a group of philosophers disputing about the production of the *lapis philosophorum*. See J. Telle (1992) for a complete bibliographic information about manuscript copies and printed editions of the *Rosarium*.

2 Andres Cafferata's work was influenced by the French psychoanalyst, Jacques Lacan, and the Argentinian psychoanalyst, David Liberman's work on psychoanalysis and language.

3 Postmodernism de-emphasises the hierarchy implicit in modern psychotherapies. Additionally, the postmodern therapies tend to elicit clients as co-creators and co-facilitators of their life narratives in the therapy process. Clients organise and give meaning to their experience through the storying of experience. In performing their stories, clients are expressing selected aspects of their lived experience (White & Epston, 1990).

4 In America, Joseph Reyher's *Emergent-uncovering method* (1977), which is a psychoanalytic imagery-based approach that has no links to RED, believes that valuable insight is gained by the patient through ongoing imagery even in the absence of any interpretation by the therapist.

Conclusion

Jung (2009) ended *The Red Book* with an unfinished 1959 epilogue with a final word that is the noun *Möglichkeit*, which in German means possibility. This work explores possibilities by looking for connections from both a historical and a theoretical perspective. The main highlights of this work include the historical account of the epistolary relationship between Jung and Desoille of March 22, 1938, and the finding of Desoille's first book in Jung's personal library in Kusnacht, which is proof that Jung had heard of Robert Desoille and that Desoille wanted to correspond with Jung. The integration of RED and active imagination is something which Desoille wished Jung to have done. In fact, on June 9, 1939, Desoille in a letter to his Swiss friend Adolphe Ferriere laments *"Je le regrette, car appliqués par lui les moyens, que j'ai indiques feraient merveille/*I regret that if Jung had applied the means that I indicated it would have been marvellous" (AdF/C/1/18). Furthermore, the correspondence between other European imaginative therapeutic practitioners and Jung, such as that of Carl Happich, Marc Guillerey, Hanscarl Leuner and Alfred Wolfsohn, has also shed interesting insights on guided imaginative therapeutic approaches that were trying to dialogue with analytical psychology and which Jung seemed to have preferred to sideline from his references.

This work also creates a filiation map of the common collaborators, friends and acquaintances of both Jung and Desoille, which brings out interesting connections previously unaccounted for in the historical development of imaginative psychotherapy in the twentieth century. The key figure amongst these collaborators of both Jung and Desoille is the psychoanalyst Charles Baudouin. Through the *Institute of Psychogagy and Psychotherapy* in Geneva, as well as through the main journal of the Institute, namely *Action et Pensée*, Baudouin seems to have been central in bringing the two psychotherapy schools together in France and Switzerland. This book also manages to trace those practitioners who had studied with Desoille and trained in the RED method before they trained as Jungians, as well as identify key French Jungians who collaborated with Desoillians in the 60s. Such findings help to bring out the inclusive spirit of some French Jungians who collaborated with those Desoillians who did not want their theory to become Freudian. It also helps to debunk the myth, at least in France and Romandy, that Jungians were insular and avoided other approaches. In fact, these findings also throw important light on the historical development of analytical psychology in these countries in the first half of the twentieth century.

This work has also managed to bring together Desoillian practitioners who stopped collaborating with each other soon after Desoille's death. Fifty years later, this work created an impetus for post-Desoillians of different denominations to come together again. This was possible through an international conference on waking dream therapy which I organised under the auspices of *The Malta Depth psychological Association*, S.I.S.P.I., Italy and the French Embassy in Malta, in May 2014. The conference also saw the launch of the *International Network for the Study of Waking Dream Therapy (I.N.S.W.D.T.)*,[1] which augurs well for more visibility and possible contacts and connections to emerge.[2]

This book also questions the Jungian notion of free imagination in active imagination both from historical sources and from a clinical perspective. It argues that an element of guidance is always present when active imagination is carried out in the therapy itself while RED is not as directive as it is made out to be. In the proposed framework, the therapist not only witnesses but actively facilitates the patient to get in touch with unconscious material. The framework emphasises the principles of facilitation, exploration, expression, holding, reciprocity, affective resonance and communicable meaning. This approach can offer practical ideas to Jungian practitioners of how to use active imagination in the therapy session. This framework fits in within a mytho-poetic therapeutic approach where analysis co-operates with poetic-imaginative reflection. The practice framework also adds an experiential approach of movement, characteristic of RED, besides one of dialogue which is usually associated with active imagination. I intend to develop this clinical practice framework of a RED-based approach to active imagination into a full therapeutic model, which I would like to refer to as "Imaginative Movement Therapy" (I.M.T.). Once the framework is developed into a new therapeutic model, its procedures, processes and outcomes have to be studied both qualitatively and quantitatively. Such studies would help to validate the method as an efficient treatment method for psychological problems with different client groups.

Further directions

Although the historical research in this work is extensive, it is not conclusive. It can continue to be deepened as new documents emerge or are found which will shed further light on other possible connections. Until now, the possible heirs of Desoille (the grand children of Desoille's brother) have not yet been traced. Unfortunately, during the time I have been developing this work (2009–2019), several important people whom I would have liked to interview either died or were too old to give an interview including Yvonne Arthus,[3] Dr. Richard Bevand,[4] Dr. Jean Nadal[5] and Dr. Jean Claude Benoit.[6] Furthermore, the correspondence of the French philosopher Gaston Bachelard is not yet accessible to the public, due to a family court case, and important information about the contacts he had with Desoille, and possibly with Jung, is thus unavailable (one letter of Jung to Bachelard of December 12, 1938 was traced at the E.T.H. Jung archives in Zurich – Hs 1056: 7186). Similarly the archives[7] of the main Desoillian school in Paris, i.e., G.I.R.E.P., were not accessible when I made contact to visit them, since they were in the process of changing location. Moreover, the correspondence between the prominent late French Jungian analyst Elie Humbert and Carl Jung was not accessible as it is remains classified by the E.T.H./ archives. This might contain important links and information during the conflict of the French Society of Analytical Psychology and the Charles Baudouin Institute. Another challenge was faced in the archives of the *Insitute Metapsychique*, in Paris, where the documents are not digitalised and thus more difficult to carry extensive research on. In fact, there could be documents that throw light on the Desoille brothers as well as other possible Jungian connections. The same holds for the Roberto Assagioli archives in Florence, which possibly provide links between psychosynthesis, analytical psychology and RED.

Research implications

In recent years, the function of imagination has regained respectability amongst psychological practitioners. In addition, the use of imagery as a therapeutic agent by cognitive behaviourists has increased considerably (Gilbert, 2010; Hackmann, Bennett-Levy & Holmes, 2011). However, this could not be said of the Jungian community until quite recently, with the publication of *The Red Book*. The French Jungian analyst Elie Humbert, in 1971, underlined the dwindling popularity of active imagination. This was also highlighted by another Jungian, August Cwik (1995), who saw the influence of the clinical/developmental school and its focus on the transference-counter-transference over-ride active imagination. The latter seems to have suffered the same fate of a loss in popularity as dream interpretation did in the classical Freudian approach (Kernberg, 1993).

The lack of popularity of active imagination proves that there is a strong need to present guidelines of how to practise active visual imagination in the therapy session itself. Even though Kast (1988, 2014) has written some case studies, she does not present a unified framework of how to practise it. The practice framework presented in this book demonstrates how the therapist can aid the patient to go deeper into an altered state of consciousness in order to facilitate ego-receptivity. Furthermore, it offers support to the patient's weak ego, which might be threatened by overwhelming emotions. Transference and counter-transference are also included in the framework, thus responding to the criticism of the developmental school (Fordham, 1967).

Furthermore, the practice framework of a RED-based approach to active imagination which can be developed into a full psychotherapeutic method which I call "Imaginative Movement Therapy" (I.M.T.) can be promoted and included amongst the Jungian expressive arts modalities which derive from Jung's active imagination, such as art therapy, drama therapy, dance/movement therapy, play and sand-play therapy. This model would give the visual approach of doing active imagination a proper framework in the expressive arts. The word "movement" in the title, besides referring to both the explorative movement and resting of the imaginal ego in the imaginative landscape, refers to the fact that when we visualise or imagine, we also stimulate the neuromuscular circuitry, thus engaging a body response even when lying down. Furthermore, the word "movement" also refers to this form of therapy as being an action-oriented therapy. Weiner (1999) uses the latter term to describe expressive therapies as "action therapies." Imaginative movement therapy would complement and also enrich drama therapy as well as movement therapeutic approaches of a Jungian perspective given that both oneiric drama, and oneiric and somatic movement are key elements of the RED-based active imagination framework.

Unfortunately, the separation of the expressive arts, including the RED-based active imagination with its visual emphasis, provokes a corresponding split within the psyche since thought and emotions are constantly interacting with and combining different modes of perception. The truth is that as we have already seen, we can experience imagination with any and all of our senses: sight, hearing, bodily sensations and movements, smell and taste. In fact, if therapy is to engage life, it must be open to the multiplicity of the psyche and its multi-sensory expressions. This is even more so since persons differ in the vividness of their imagery and in perceptual capacity, excelling in one or more sensory modes over another. Most individuals are good at more than one type and rarely think in one exclusive sensory mode, while a few seldom form representation in any sensory mode. The reasons could boil down to constitutional, environmental and cultural experience.

The hybridised-integrated practice framework of a RED-based approach to active imagination brings up the issue of "primacy" and consequently one of identity. The imaginative movement therapist would probably find her- or himself in a difficult position, neither purely in Jungian territory nor on the Desoillian side. This composite framework is made up of distinctly different components, each of which maintains its individual identity within the practice framework. In remaining committed to a plural perspective, I avoid any attempt to synthesise the two therapeutic methods and thus develop a hybridised-integrated framework instead. In the creation of a hybridised-integrated format, the coming together of different elements creates a transformative energy, which brings forth an innovative approach to active imagination. However, until the new therapeutic modality of "Imaginative Movement Therapy" begins a history of its own, the question of recognition and legitimacy is bound to remain.

This book also brings forward the need for analytical psychology to dialogue with and be influenced by other schools of thought. It has shown how Jung guarded his approach and couched it in a way that looked unique and could not be compared to other European imaginative approaches. At a time when depth psychology is less popular than it was 50 years ago, it is even more important that analytical psychology opens its doors to other approaches, such as RED. Active imagination has been applied and absorbed by expressive arts therapies and it can also be integrated with other psychotherapies of different modalities which use the imagination in their work. The same can be said of RED, which despite being considerably known in France has kept a low profile in other parts of the world. This could be because of the lack of RED literature in English which makes the directed waking dream method less understood. Furthermore, the lack of interest amongst RED French practitioners to market their approach on an international level does not help either. Ironically, Desoille himself had also shown interest in lucid dreaming and he had written a preface to the 1964 re-issue of the book of Hervey de Saint-Denys "*Les Rêves et les Moyens de les Diriger*/Dreams and How to Direct Them" (Tchou, 1964). From a Jungian perspective, the work of Hall and Brylowski (1991), who tried to see the implications of lucid dreaming to active imagination, can continue to open new avenues amongst these two methods.

This book also puts into the foreground Robert Desoille, an almost forgotten figure in the history of European psychotherapy, namely due to the increasing popularity of Lacanian psychoanalysis, the French version of psychoanalysis which dominated the scene after the Second World War until the 1960s. Lacanian psychoanalysis overshadowed the psychotherapeutic dialogue which Desoille started in France with different therapeutic approaches in the 1940s, where RED was very much visible. His reserved nature, which kept him back from promoting his method on a large scale, together with his Pavlovian turn towards the end of his life at a time when psychoanalysis was becoming increasingly popular, especially in France, signified his exit from the therapeutic centre stage. Nonetheless, there is a big need to publish a full appreciation of Desoille's work, in terms not only of his method which makes him an important pioneer in imaginative psychotherapy, but of him as a serious scientific experimental researcher who put to the test graphical recording instruments which were invented by engineers and widely used in medicine and experimental research (Brain, 2008). In fact, his research endeavours put him close to the physiological movement of the nineteenth and twentieth centuries and he brilliantly applied the ideas of Charles Henry and Gustav Fechner on aesthetic physiology to his waking dream method. He also applied the result of psycho-physiologists like Hans Berger on waking and sleep states to his method. Desoille's interest in research seems to run parallel to the interest shown by the young Jung as a medical doctor at the Burghozli hospital in the early years of the twentieth century.[8] The information gathered on Robert Desoille alone, including his personal life, while carrying out this work, merits a book on its own.

Furthermore, this work continues with the tradition of historical revisionism conducted by Jungians, such as the initiative taken by Jungian analyst Prof. Andrew Samuels vis-à-vis Jung's anti-Semitic comments in the 1930s. This effort led to the correction of some of Jung's theories about Jews lacking a culture of their own, which he claimed turned them into a "parasite" (Samuels, 1994). Likewise, though on a different tone, Jungians may have to acknowledge Jung's failure to acknowledge other European pioneers of imaginative therapies in his time, as well as for the hard comments made from some of his close disciples against practitioners who worked with guided imagery in order to protect their new emerging discipline of analytical psychology.

Conclusion

This book tries to put into practise Jung's quote that "Without the playing of fantasy no creative work has ever yet come to birth. The debt we owe to the play of imagination is incalculable" (Jung, 1921/1971, p. 63 [CW6, para. 93]). It re-imagines Jung's technique of active imagination itself both from a historical and from a theoretical perspective. I hope this book will provide another useful source of ideas on how to stimulate imagination in therapy for analytical psychologists, RED analysts and other therapeutic professionals, as well as offer Jungian scholars new historical perspectives on waking dream therapeutic approaches at the turn of the twentieth century. Waking dreams are indeed an important part of our European psychotherapeutic heritage, and according to Desoille (1945), they remain relevant to the teaching of the art of living, which is open to all ages.

Notes

1 www.wakingdreamtherapy.org.
2 A professor from Crete, namely Prof Anastasia-Valentine Rigas, who studied with the niece of Desoille in Paris, Dr. Monique Pellerin, has also been identified and contacted. So far, the contacts Desoille made in Japan could not be traced.
3 She was the wife of Dr. A. Arthus and died aged 106 during 2012.
4 Dr. Richard Bevand died in 2019.

5 A disciple of Desoille, interested in Jung but who later adopted RED along Freudian lines and who also taught the Jungian Christian Gaillard the RED method. In a personal communication on March 30, 2013. Gaillard explains:

> Il se trouve que j'ai eu l'expérience d'une formation à cette pratique alors que je faisais mon doctorat à Paris, et avant de m'engager dans l'analyse jungienne/It happens that I have had a training before I did my doctorate in Paris and before doing my Jungian analytic training. (my translation)

6 Dr. Jean Claude Benoit Benoit collaborated with Dr. Mario Berta in Uruguay. He died in 2018.

7 I met the person responsible for the archives of G.I.R.E.P. in 2019 and realised that they mainly hold documents related to the history of G.I.R.E.P. and not much on the earlier history.

8 Desoille's first wife, Lucie, was instrumental in introducing Desoille to waking dreams, as well as to the writing of his first two books. His second wife Mireille was also supportive in the development and teaching of Desoille's method.

Bibliography

Aboulkher-Muscat, C. (1995). *Alone with the one*. New York: ACMI Press.

Adler, G. (1957). *Etudes de psychologie jungienne. Essais sur la théorie et la pratique de l'analyse jungienne* [Studies in analytical psychology. Essay on the theory and practice of Jungian analysis]. Genève: Georg Editeurs.

Adler, G. (1961). *The living symbol: A case study in the process of individuation*. New York: Pantheon Books.

Ahsen, A. (1965). *Eidetic psychotherapy: A short introduction*. New York: Brandon House.

Aigrisse, G. (1967). Andre Virel, histoire de notre image. *Journal of Analytical Psychology, 12*(2), 175–186.

Ajuriaguerra, J. (1959). *L'Entraînement psychophysiologique par la relaxation* [Psycho- physiological training for relaxation]. Paris: Expansion scientifique.

Alexander, F., & French, M. T. (1946). *Psychoanalytic therapy*. New York: The Ronald Press Company.

Ammon, G. (Ed.). (1974). *Gruppendynamik der kreativität* [Group dynamics of creativity]. München: Kindler TB.

Anastasia, H. (2012, 1 May). Electronic communication from Dr. Hector Anastasia to author.

Andjelkovic, L., Aumage, M., Guilhot, A. M., & Pellerin, M. (1983). Intérêt du rêve éveillé dans les cures de patients psychosomatiques [Interest in waking dream in the cure of psychosomatic patients]. *Etudes Psychothérapiques, 51*(1), 7–12.

Appleton, V. (2011). Avenues of hope: Art therapy and the resolution of trauma. *Art Therapy, 18*(1), 6–13.

Aron, L. (1996). *A meeting of minds. Mutuality in psychoanalysis*. Hillsdale, NJ: Analytic Press.

Arthus, A. (1956). *Le Rêve éveillé libre* [Free waking dream]. *Action et Pensée, 1*(Mars), 8–16.

Arthus, A. (1971, Nov–Dec). Le fantastique onirique [Oneiric fantasy]. *Psychotherapies: Revue de l'Arbre Vert, 4*, 3–10.

Arzel Nadal, L. (2006). *Francoise Dolto et l'image inconsciente du corps: fondements et deplacement vers la pulsion* [Francoise Dolto and the unconscious body image: Foundations and deplacement towards the impulse]. Bruxelles: De Boeck.

Ashton, P. (2010). Music, mind and psyche. In P. Ashton & S. Bloch (Eds.), *Music and psyche: Contemporary psychoanalytic explorations* (pp. 121–142). New Orleans: Spring Journal Books.

Assagioli, R. (1959). 7th Newsletter of the Psychosynthesis Research Foundation, Inc. U.S.A. issued in September, 1959 (Retrieved from: psychosynthesisresources.com).

Austin, D. (2006). In-depth music psychotherapy. *Voices: Journal of the American Academy of Psychotherapists*, 42(2), 20–31.

Avila, T. (1979). *The interior castle* (K. Kavanaugh and O. Rodriguez, Trans.). Mahwah, NJ: Paulist Press.

Aziz, R. (1990). *C. G. Jung's psychology of religion and synchronicity*. Albany: State University of New York Press.

Azvedo-Fernandes, M. L. (1953). Aluz Azul (La lumiere bleue). Etude d'un case [Blue light. A case-study]. *O. Medico*. Porto, 79.

Bachelard, G. (1943). *L'air et les songes: essai sur l'imagination du movement* [Air and dreams: Essay on the imagination of movement]. Paris: Librairie Jose Corti.

Bachelard, G. (1948). *La terre et les rêveries de la volonté: essai sur l'imagination des forces* [The earth and the reveries of will: Essay on the imagination of forces]. Paris: Librairie Jose Corti.

Bachelard, G. (1960). *La poétique de la rêverie* [Poetics of reverie]. Paris: Presses Universitaires de France.

Bachelard, G. (1964). *The poetics of space*. New York: Orion Press.

Baier, K. (2013). Meditation im scnittfeld von psychotherapie, hochgradfreimaurerei und kirchenreform – Carl Happichs innovationen und ihr sozio kultureller context. In R. Almut-Barbara & C. Wulf (Hg.), *Meditation in religion, therapie, asthetik und bildung. Paragrana. Internationale Zeitschrift für Historische Anthropologie*, 22(2), 51–76. Berlin: Akademie Verlag.

Balzarini, G. (1985). L'Analisi immaginativa, intervista al Dr. G. Balzarini [Imaginative analysis, interview with Dr. G. Balzarini], *Synthesis, IV(7)*, Piovan Editore.

Barber, T. X. (1961). Physiological aspects of hypnosis. *Psychological Bulletin, 58*, 390–419.

Barber, T. X. (1965). Physiological effects of "hypnotic suggestions": A critical review of recent research. *Psychological Bulletin, 63*, 201–222.

Barnard, W. G. (2012). Turning into other worlds. Henri Bergson and the radio reception theory of consciousness. In A. Lefebre & M. White (Eds.), *Bergson, politics and religion* (pp. 281–298). Durham, NC: Duke University Press.

Baron, P. (1989). Fighting cancer with images. In H. Wadeson (Ed.), *Advances in art therapy* (pp. 148–168). New York: Wiley.

Barthes, R. (1989). *Sade, Fourier, Loyola,* (R. Miller, Trans.). Berkeley and Los Angeles: University of California Press.

Baudelaire, C. (1962). *Curiosités esthétiques* [Aesthetic curiosities]. Paris: Garnier.

Baudouin, C. (1920). *Suggestion et autosuggestion* [Suggestion and autosuggestion]. Neuchâtel-Paris: Delachaux & Niestlé.

Baudouin, C. (2007). *De l'instinct a l'esprit* [From the instinct to the spirit]. Paris: Editions Imago. (Originally published in 1950).

Baudouin, C. (1954, Dec). Notes sur le pouvoir regenerateur du 'rêve dirigé' [Notes on the regenerative force of the guided dream]. *Action et Pensée, 4*, 113–115.

Baudouin, C. (1963). *L'Œuvre de Jung: études et documents* [The work of Jung: Studies and documents]. Paris: Payot.

Becker, K. (2001). *Unlikely companions: C. G. Jung on the spiritual exercises of Ignatius of Loyola*. Leominister: Gracewing.

Beebe, J. (1981). *Film as active imagination*. Recorded seminar, C. G. Jung Institute of San Francisco, October 10–11, 1981.

Beebe, J. (2010). Psychotherapy and the aesthetic attitude. *Journal of Analytical Psychology*, 55(2), 168–186.

Benoit, J. C. (1973). Le *rêve éveillé thérapique* [The therapeutic waking dream]. In P. Sivadon, *Traite de Psychologie medicale, Tome 2, La rencontre thérapique* (pp. 185–195). Paris: Presses Universitaires de France.

Berdach, E., & Bakan, P. (1967). Body position and free recall of early memories. *Psychotherapy: Therapy, Research and Practice*, 4, 101–102.

Berge, A. (1974). *Les psychotherapies* (2nd ed). [Psychotherapies]. Paris: Presses Universitaires de France.

Berger, J. (2009). The eaters and the eaten. In J. Berger (Ed.), *Why look at animals?* (pp. 61–69). London: Penguin. (Originally published in 1976).

Bergson, H. (1912). *Schopferische entwicklung* [Creative evolution]. Jena: E. Diederichs. (Originally published in French as *L'Évolution créatrice* in 1907).

Bergson, H. (1928). *Die seelische energie* [Mind-energy]. Jena: E. Diederichs. (Orginally published in French as *L'Énergie spirituelle* in 1919).

Bergson, H. (1932). *Les deux sources de la morale et de la religion*. [The two sources of morality and religion]. Paris: Universitaires de France.

Bernsteirn, S. J. (2005). *Living in the borderland: The evolution of consciousness and the challenge of healing trauma*. East Sussex: Routledge.

Berta, M. (1962). Reve eveille lisergico dirigado. [Directed lysergic waking dream]. *Revista de Psiquiatria del Uruguay*, 27, 159–180.

Berta, M. (1999). *L'epreuve d'anticipation. Test de l'imaginaire personnel*. [The anticipation trial. Test of the personal imagination]. Ramonville Saint-Agne: Editons Eres.

Berta, M. (2000). *Les images qui guerrisent. Le "Rêve éveillé dirigé" de Robert Desoille* [The images that heal. The directed waking dream of Robert Desoille]. Texte inédit. Montevideo.

Berta, M. (2001). *La tercera revolucion en psicoterapia – Psicoactivation: Teoria y practica sistemico-evolutivas* [The third revolution in psychotherapy – Psychoactivation: Theory and practice of evolutionary systems]. Conferencia pronunciade en la Academia Nacional de Medicina el 16 agosto de 2001. Presentacion del academic Prof. Dr. Daniel Murguia. Montevideo: El Toboso.

Berta, M., & Anastasia, H. (2002). *La era de la imaginacion simbolica* [The era of symbolic imagination]. Montevideo: El Toboso.

Berti, A. (1988). *Roberto Assagioli: Profilo biografico degli anni di formazione* [Roberto Assagioli: Biographical profile of the formative years]. Firenze: Istituto di Psicosintesi.

Best, S., & Kellner, D. (1991). *Post-modern theory: Critical interrogations*. New York: Guilford Press.

Bevand, R. (1961). Traitement d'une phobie par le R.E.D. [Treatment of phobia with R.E.D.]. *Action et Pensée*, Geneve, *XXXV11*(1), 12–17.

Binswanger, L., & Foucault, M. (1993). *Dream and existence*. K. Hoeller (Ed.). Atlantic Highlands, NJ: Humanities Press. (Originally published as *Traum und Existenz* by L. Bisnwanger in 1930).

Bion, W. R. (1962). A theory of thinking. *International Journal of Psychoanalysis*, 43, 306–310.

Bishop, P. (2012). Jung's red book and its relation to aspects of German Idealism. *Journal of Analytical Psychology, 57*, 335–363.

Blajan-Marcus, S., & Raynaud, A. (1997). *De memoire de psychoanalyste. Quarante ans d'experience Clinique* [Memoirs of a psychoanalyst. Forty years of clinical experience]. Paris: Editions Imago.

Bloch, S. (2007). Music as dreaming: Absence and the Emergence of the Auditory Symbol – Stephen Bloch. In P. W. Ashton (Ed.), *Evocations of Absence: Multidisciplinary Perspectives on Void States.* New Orleans: Spring Journal Books.

Bloom, H. (1973). *The anxiety of influence. A theory of poetry.* New York: Oxford University Press.

Bonny, L. H. (1978). *Facilitating GIM sessions.* Salina, KS: Bonny Foundation.

Bordwell, D., & Thompson, K. (2008). *Film art: An introduction,* 8th ed. Boston: McGraw Hill.

Bosnak, R. (1986). *A little course in dreams.* Bostan, MA: Shambala.

Bosnak, R. (2007). *Embodiment: Creative imagination in medicine, art and travel.* London: Routledge.

Bourdieu, P. (2000). *Esquisse d'une théorie de la pratique* [Outline of a theory of practice]. Paris: Seuil. (Originally published in 1972).

Bovensiepen, G. (2002). Symbolic attitude and reverie. Problems of symbolisation in children and adolescents. *Journal of Analytical Psychology, 47*(2), 241–257.

Bovet, P. (1936, Jan 10). *Letter of Pierre Bovet to Charles Baudouin* (Ms fr 5954 f 6). Département des manuscrits, Bibliothèque de Genève.

Brain, R. M. (2008). The pulse of modernism: Experimental physiology and aesthetic avant-gardes circa 1900. *Studies in History and Philosophy of Science, 39*(3), 393–417.

Bres, M., & Pellerin, M. (2005). *La Revue de Psychosynthese,* [Review of psychosynthesis]. *17,* Juin, 7–10.

Britton, R. (1989). The missing link: Parental sexuality in the Oedipus complex. In J. Steiner (Ed.), *The Oedipus complex today: Clinical implications* (pp. 83–101). London: Karnac.

Bromberg, P. (2001). *Standing in the spaces: Essays on clinical process, trauma, and dissociation.* Hillsdale, NJ: Analytic Press.

Brome, V. (1978). *Jung: Man and myth.* London: Macmillan.

Bronner, S. E. (1992). *Moments of decision: Political history and the crises of radicalism.* New York: Routledge.

Brower, M. B. (2010). *Unruly spirits. The science of psychic phenomena in modern France.* Urbana, Chicago and Springfield: University of Illinois Press.

Brutsche, P. (2011). The Red Book in the context of Jung's paintings. *Jung Journal: Culture & Psyche, 5*(3), 8–25.

Butler, C. (2003). *Post-modernism: A very short introduction.* New York: Oxford University Press.

Callois, R. (1970). *L'ecriture des pierres.* [The writing stones]. Genève: Editions d'Art Albert Skira.

Cambray, J. (2001). Enactments and amplifications. *Journal of Analytical Psychology, 46*(2), 275–305.

Cane, F. (1951). *The artist in each of us.* New York: Pantheon Books.

Carere-Comes, T. (2001). Assimilative and accommodative integration: The basic dialectics. *Journal of Psychotherapy Integration, 11*(1), 105–115.

Carotenuto, A. (1985). *The vertical labyrinth. Individuation in Jungian psychology.* Toronto: Inner City Books.

Carter, L. (2010). Countertransference and intersubjectivity. In M. Stein (Ed.), *Jungian psychoanalysis: Working in the spirit of C. G. Jung* (pp. 201–212). Chicago, IL: Open Court.

Cary, P. (2000). *Augustine's invention of the inner self.* Oxford: Oxford University Press.

Case, C. (2000). Our lady of the queen: Journeys around the maternal object. In A. Gilroy & G. McNeilly (Eds.), *The changing shape of art therapy: New developments in the theory and practise* (pp. 15–54). London and Philadelphia: Jessica Kingsley Publisher.

Caslant, E. (1937). *Méthode de dévelopment des facultés supra-normales* (3rd. Ed.) [Method for the development of supra-normal faculties]. Paris: Editions Jean Meyer. (Originally published in 1927).

Cifali, M. (1995). Les débuts de la psychoanalyse en Suisse [The debut of psychoanalysis in Switzerland]. *Nervure, Journal de Psychiatrie, 8,* 10–17.

Champernowne, I. (1969). Art therapy as an adjunct to psychotherapy. *Inscape, 1,* 1–10.

Champernowne, I. (1971). Art and therapy: An uneasy partnership. *Inscape,* 3, 1–14.

Charet, F. X. (1993). *Spiritualism and the foundations of C. G. Jung's psychology.* Albany: State University of New York Press.

Chiore, V. (2004). *Il poeta, l'alchimista, il demone* [The poet, the alchemist and the devil]. Genova: Il Melangolo.

Chodorow, J. (1995). Dance/movement and body experience in analysis. In M. Stein (Ed.), *Jungian Analysis* (2nd Ed.) (pp. 391–404). Chicago, IL: Open Court.

Chodorow, J. (1997). *C. G. Jung on active imagination. Key readings selected and introduced by Joan Chodorow.* London: Routledge.

Choisy, M. (1949). *Yogas et psychoanalyse [Yoga and psychoanalysis].* Geneve: Editions du Mont-Blanc.

Clarke, J. J. (1992). *In search of Jung.* London: Routledge.

Clarke, J. J. (1994). *Jung and Eastern thought.* London: Routledge.

Clark, L. P. (1925). The phantasy method of analyzing narcissistic neuroses. *Psychoanalytic Review, X111,* 225–232.

Coleman, W. (2006). Imagination and the imaginary. *Journal of Analytical Psychology, 51*(1), 21–41.

Coleridge, S. T. (1907). *Biographia literaria.* London: Oxford University Press. (Originally published in 1817).

Colette, F., & M. Mesnil. (2009). L'introduction du RED dans des séances de psychothérapies de groupe d'adolescents dyssociaux. *Imaginaire et Inconscient,* 24, 47–63.

Conger, J. P. (2005). *Jung and Reich: The body as shadow.* Berkeley, CA: North Atlantic Books.

Connolly, A. (2014). Alchemy in 'The Red Book' of C. G. Jung. *Quaderni di Cultura Junghiana, 3,* 101–107.

Cooper, M., & McLeod, J. (2007). A pluralistic framework for counselling and psychotherapy: Implications for research. *Counselling and Psychotherapy Research, 7,* 135–143.

Copleston, F. C. (1958). *History of philosophy, volume IV: Descartes to Leibniz.* Mahwah, NJ: Paulist Press.

Corbin, H. (1972). Mundus imaginalis, or the imaginary and the imaginal. *Spring,* 1–19. Dallas: Spring Publications.

Corbin, H. (1983). Theophanies and mirrors: Idols or icons? (trans: Pratt, J. A., & Donohue, A. K.). *Spring: An Annual of Archetypal Psychology and Jungian Thought, 198,* 1–2.

Corbishley, T. (1963). *The spiritual exercises of Saint Ignatius of Loyola.* New York: P. J. Kennedy & Sons.

Cosgrove, D. (1999). Introduction. In D. Cosgrove (Ed.), *Mappings* (pp. 1–23). London: Reaktion Books.

Coué, É. (1922). *La maîtrise de soi-même par l'autosuggestion consciente (Autrefois: De la suggestion et de ses applications)* [Self-mastery through conscious auto-suggestion (Or: Suggestions and their applications]. P Nancy: Société Lorraine de psychologie appliqué.

Crowley, A. (1909). *Liber 777.* London: The Walter Scott Publishing Co., Ltd.

Cwik, J. A. (1991). Active imagination as imaginal play space. In N. Schwartz-Salant & M. Stein (Eds.), *Liminality and transitional phenomena* (pp. 99–114). Wilmette, IL: Chiron.

Cwik, J. A. (1995). Active imagination: Synthesis in analysis. In M. Stein (Ed.), *Jungian Analysis* (pp. 136–169). Chicago and La Salle, IL: Open Court.

Cwik, J. A. (2006). The art of the tincture: Analytical supervision. *Journal of Analytical Psychology, 51*(2), 209–225.

Dalbiez, R. (1941). *Psychoanalytical method and the doctrine of Freud* (T. F. Lindsay, Trans.). London: Longmans, Green & Co. (Originally published in 1936).

Dallett, J. (1982). Active imagination: Synthesis in analysis. In M. Stein (Ed.), *Jungian Analysis* (2nd ed.) (pp. 173–191). La Salle, IL: Open Court.

Dallett, J. (2008). *Listening to the rhino: Violence and healing in a scientific age.* New York: Pleasure Boat Studio: A Literary Press.

Dallet, T., Rifkind, G., & Terry, K. (1993). *The three voices of art therapy.* London: Routledge.

Daniels, A. B. (2014). *Jungian crime scene analysis: An imaginal investigation.* London: Karnac Books.

Daudet, L. (1926). *Le rêve éveillé: étude sur la profondeur de l'esprit* [The waking dream: A study on the depth of the spirit]. Paris: Grasset.

David, M. (1973). Jung e la cultura francese [Jung and the French culture]. *Rivista di Psicologia Analitica, 4*(2), 463–504.

Davidson, D. (1966). Transference as active imagination. *Journal of Analytical Psychology, 11,* 135–145.

De Baudot, A. (1889–1890). Sur les reformes à introduire dans l'education de l'architecte [On the reforms of the education in architecture]. *Encyclopedie d'architecture,* t. 2, 6–7.

De Certeau, M. (1984). *The practise of everyday life* (S. Rendall, Trans.). Berkeley: University of California Press.

Delpech, J. L. (1967). Essai sur la genèse de la méthode du *"Rêve éveillé dirigé en psychothérapie"* de Robert Desoille [Essay on the beginnings of the directed waking dream method in psychotherapy of Robert Desoille]. *En Hommage a*

Monsieur Robert Desoille: Bulletin de la Société de recherché psychotherapiques de langue francaise, V, 1, Mars, 5–10.

De Mijolla, A. (2012). *La France et Freud (Tome 1, 1946–1953) Une penible renaissance*. Paris: Presses Universitaires de France.

Deniau., Desoille, R., Fayol., Renaud., & Virel. (1966). Transfert et contre-transfert dans le rêve éveillé dirigé [Transference and counter-transference in the directed waking dream]. *Groupe d'etude du Rêve éveillé dirigé, colloque du 26 Fevrier, 1966. Société de recerches psychothérapiques de langue Francaise*, 2, 63–66.

Derrida, J. (1978). *Writing and difference* (A. Bass, Trans.). Chicago, IL: University of Chicago Press.

Descamps, M. A. (1985). Les contes de Perrault et l'analyse Rêve-éveillé [Perrault's fairy-tales and the waking dream analysis]. *Etudes Psychothérapiques*, 60(2), 95–102.

Descamps, M. A. (2004). *La psychanalyse spiritualiste* [Spiritualistic psychoanalysis]. Paris: Desclée de Brouwer.

Desoille, R. (1928, Jan–Feb.). Contribution a l'etude des effets psychologiques du Peyotl [A contribution for the study of the psychological effects of Peyotl]. *Revue Metapsychique*, 1, 37–58.

Desoille, R. (1928). Rapport de M. Desoille, Ingenieur – Un lien existe-t-il entre les etats de conscience et les phenomenes electro-magnetiques? [Report of Mr. Desoille, Engineer – Is there a link between the conscious state and the electro-magnetic phenomena]. *En Compte Rendu du 111eme Congres International de Recherches Psychiques, A Paris Septembre – Octobre, 1927, pp. 56–68*. Paris: Institute Metapsychique International.

Desoille, R. (1930, Nov–Dec). A propos de l'hynpotisme [On hynosis]. *Revue Metapsychique*, 6, 502–506.

Desoille, R. (1932, Nov–Dec). De quelques conditions auxquelles il faut satisfaire pour réussir des expériences de téléphathie provoquée [What are the conditions one has to satisfy to be able to experience induced telepathy]. *Revue Metapsychique*, 6, 410–417.

Desoille, R. (1931, Mai). Une méthode rationnelle pour l'exploration du subconscient [A rational method for the exploration of the sub-conscious]. *Action et Pensée*, 5, 241–247.

Desoille, R. (1938). *Exploration de l'affectivité subconsciente par la méthode du rêve éveillé: sublimation et acquisitions psychologiques* [An exploration of the subconscious emotions through the waking dream method: Sublimation and psychological acquistions]. Paris: J.L.L. D'Artrey.

Desoille, R. (1945). *Le rêve éveillé en psychothérapie: Essai sur la fonction de régulation de l'inconscient collectif* [The waking dream in psychotherapy: Essay on the regulatory function of the collective unconscious]. Paris: Presses universitaires de France.

Desoille, R. (1948). Le rêve éveillé et la filmologie [The waking dream and filmology]. *Revue Internationale de filmologie*, 1, 3–4, Octobre.

Desoille, R. (1948). Le rêve éveillé dirigé et la creation artistique [The waking dream and artistic creation]. *Arts Lettres*, 11, 53–55.

Desoille. R. (1955). *Introduction a une psychotherapie rationelle* [An introduction to a rational psychotherapy]. Paris: Editions l'Arche.

Desoille. R. (1956). Liberte et direction dans le Rêve éveillé [Liberty and directivity in the waking dream]. *Action et Pensée, 1(Mars)*, 16–21.

Desoille, R. (1957). Le rêve éveillé dirige comme method d'exploration et de cure psychologique [The waking dream as a method of psychological exploration and cure]. *Archives Hospitalieres et Revue Science et Sante Reunies, 8,* 221–229.

Desoille, R. (1960). Tenth newsletter issued in July, 1960 by the Psychosynthesis research Foundantion, Inc., USA. (Retrieved from: http://www.psychosynthesis-resources.com/NieuweBestanden/NewslettersPRF.pdf)

Desoille, R. (1961). *Théorie et pratique du Rêve Éveillé Dirigé* [Theory and praticse of the directed waking dream]. Genève: Éditions du Mont-Blanc.

Desoille, R. (1962). Rêve éveillé dirigé et LSD 25 [Directed waking dream and LSD 25]. *Groupe du Rêve éveillé dirigé, Bulletin de la Société de Recherches Psychothérapiques de Langue Francaise,* 1(3), 25–29.

Desoille, R. (1964a). 22nd newsletter issued in February of 1964 by the Psychosynthesis Research Foundation, Inc., U.S.A. (Retrieved from: http://www.psychosynthesisresources.com/NieuweBestanden/NewslettersPRF.pdf)

Desoille, R. (1964b). Vers un nouvelle clef du songes [Towards a new way through dreams]. In C. Tchou (Ed.), Hervey de Saint-Denys, *Les Rêves et les Moyens de les Diriger.* Paris: Bibliothèque du Merveilleux.

Desoille, R. (1964c). Compte-rendu d'activite – Reunion du Novembre, 1963. [Minutes of activity – November reunion, 1963]. *Groupe du Rêve éveillé dirigé, Bulletin de la Société de Recherches Psychothérapiques de Langue Francaise.*

Desoille, R. (1966a). *The directed daydream* (F. Haronian, Trans.). New York: Psychosynthesis Research Foundation.

Desoille, R. (1966b). Preface. In G. Lanfranchi (Ed.), *"De la vie intérieure à la vie de relation"* [Preface to the "Interior life and the life of relating"] (pp. 17–19). Editions sociales.

Desoille, R. (1971). *Marie-Clotilde. Une psychothérapie par le Rêve Éveillé Dirigé* [Marie-Clothilde. A directed waking dream psychotherapy]. Paris, Payot.

Desoille, R. (1973). *Entretiens sur le Rêve Éveillé Dirigé en psychothérapie* [Interviews on the directed waking dream in psychotherapy]. Paris: Payot.

Desoille, R., & Delaville, M. (1929). Le métabolisme de base tel qu'il a été défini par Magnus-Lévy représente-t-il vraiment la dépense minima d'entretien de l'organisme? [To what extent does the basic metabolism as defined by Magnus-Levy represent the minimum maintenance expenditure of the organism]. *Comptes rendus des séances de l'academie des sciences – Juillet – Decembre, 1930.*

Desoille, R., Fayol, Y., Leuret, S., & Violet-Conil, M. (1950). *Psychoanalyse et rêve éveillé dirigé* [Psychoanalysis and directed waking dream]. Bar-le-duc: Comte-Jacquet.

De Vriese, E. (1971). Psychotherapie d'un adulte begue [Psychotherapy of a man who stutters]. *Etudes Psychotherapiques,* 3(1), 45–56.

DeWaal, E. (1993). *The spiritual journey. Word & spirit – A monastic review.* Petersham: MA: St. Bede's Publications, p. 49.

Dick, B. (1998). *The oxford group and alchoholics anonymous. A design for living that works.* Kihei III, Paradise Research Publications, Inc.

Dieckmann, H. (1979). Active imagination. In H. Dieckmann (Ed.), *Methods in analytical psychology: An introduction* (pp. 183–192), Wilmette: Chiron Publications.

Dieckmann, H. (1986). *Twice-told tales: The psychological use of fairy tales.* Wilmette, IL: Chiron Publications.

Dieckmann, H. (1997). Fairy-tales in psychotherapy. *Journal of Analytical Psychology, 42*(2), 253–268.

Donfrancesco, F. (2009). *Soul-making: Interweaving art and analysis.* London: Karnac Books.

Dorb, S. L. (2012). *Reading the Red Book: An interpretive guide to C. G. Jung's Liber Novus.* New Orleans, LA. Spring Journal Books.

Dorkel, O., Lambert, J., & Virel, A. (2010). *La decentration* [Decentration]. Paris: Editions de l' Arbre Vert.

Douglas, C. (1993). *Translate this darkness. The life of Christina Morgan.* New York: Simon & Schuster.

Downing, C. (1993). *Gods in our midst: Mythological images of the masculine: A woman's view.* New York: Crossroads.

Downing, J. N. (2004). Psychotherapy practice in a pluralistic world: Philosophical and moral dilemmas. *Journal of Psychotherapy Integration, 14*(2), 123–148.

Draaisma, D. (2000). *Metaphors of memory: A history of ideas about the mind.* Cambridge: Cambridge University Press.

Duarte, A. (2007). *El ensueno dirigido de Desoille – Manual* [The directed waking dream of Desoille – A manual]. Montevideo: SUED.

Dufour, R. (1962). Rorschach et R.E.D. [Rorschach and R.E.D.]. *Bulletin de la Société Francaise du Rorshach et des methods projectives,* Avril, 13–14, 59–66.

Dufour, R. (1978). *Ecouter le rêve* [Listen to the dream]. *Paris: Laffont.*

Durand, G. (1999). *The anthropological structures of the imaginary.* Virginia: Boombana Publications. (Originally published in 1960).

Edinger, E. F. (1984). *The creation of consciousness. Jung's myth for modern man.* Canada: Inner City Books.

Edinger, F. E. (1985). *Anatomy of the psyche: Alchemical symbolism in psychotherapy.* La Salle, IL: Open Court.

Edwards, M. (2010). In Malcolm Learmonth & Karen Huckvale (Eds.), *A Jungian circumambulation of art and therapy – Ornithology for the birds.* Exeter: Insider Art.

Eggis, H. (1960). *Essai sur le rêve vêcu en psychotherapie (la Methode Guillerey)* [Essay on the experienced dream in psychotherapy (The Guillerey Method)]. These Médecine, Université de Lausanne, Zurich, Orell Fussli.

Eliade, M. (1948). Durohana and the "Waking Dream." In K. Bharatalyer (Ed.), *Art and Thought: Issued in honour of Ananada K. Coomaraswamy on the occasion of his 70th birthday* (pp. 209–213). London: Luzac.

Eliade, M. (1951). *Le Chamanisme et les techniques archaïques de l'extase* [Shamanism and archaic techniques of ecstasy]. Paris: Payot.

Eliade, M. (1952). *Images et simboles* [Images and symbols]. Paris: Gallimard.

Eliade, M. (1954). *The myth of the eternal return* (Willard R. Task, Trans.). New York: Pantheon Books.

Eliade, M. (1954). *Le Yoga. Immortalité et liberté.* Paris: Librairie Payot.

Eliade, M. (1959). *The sacred and the profane. The nature of religion* (W. Task, Trans.). New York: Harcourt, Brace and World.

Eliade, M. (1977). Eliade's interview for 'Combat'. In W. McGuire & R. F. C. Hull (Eds.), *C. G. Jung Speaking – Interviews and encounters* (pp. 225–234). Princeton, NJ: Princeton University Press. (Originally published in 1952).

Eliade, M. (1982). *Ordeal by labyrinth: Conversations with Claude-Henri Rocquet* (D. Coltman, Trans.). Chicago, IL: University of Chicago Press.

Eliade, M. (1990). *Journal 1 (1944–1955)* (L. Ricketts, Trans.). Chicago, IL: University Chicago Press. (Originally published in French in 1973).

Ellenberger, F. H. (1970). *The discovery of the unconscious. The history and evolution of dynamic psychiatry.* New York: Basic Books.

Epstein, G. (1989). *Healing visualizations: Creating health through imagery.* New York: Bantam Books.

Epstein, G. (1994). *Healing into immortality: A new spiritual medicine of healing stories and imagery.* New York: Bantam Books.

Epstein, G. (2000). *Waking dream therapy: Unlocking the secrets of self through dreams and the imagination.* New York: Acmi Press.

Evans, R. J. (1997). *In defence of history.* London: Granta.

Evrard, R. (2016). *La légende de l'esprit: enquête sur 150 ans de parapsychologie.* [The legend of the spirit: An enquiry into 150 years of parapsychology]. Paris: Trajectoire.

Fabre, N. (1971). *Olivier. Psychothérapie d'un enfant de huit ans sans rêve éveillé dirigé* [Olivier. Psychotherapy with an eight year old without directed waking dream]. *Etudes Psychothérapiques, 5*(4), 139–150.

Fabre, N. (1973). *Le triangle brisé, Trois récits de psychothérapie d'enfant à qui il manque l'un des deux parents* [The broken triangle, three psychotherapy narratives about a child who lacked one of the parents]. Paris: Payot.

Fabre, N. (1974). Attitude RED sans RED dans une cure d'enfant [A RED attitude without RED in the cure of a child]. *Etudes Psychothérapiques, 12–13*(2/3), 105–112.

Fabre, N. (1979a). "Enfant cassés" en psychothérapie ["Broken children" in psychotherapy]. *Etudes Psychothérapiques, 38*(4), 301–306.

Fabre, N. (1979b). *Avant l'oedipe* [Before oedipus]. Paris: Masson Editeur.

Fabre, N. (1982). *L'enfant e le rêve-éveillé: Une approache psychothérapique de l'enfant.* [The infant and the waking dream. A child psychotherapy approach]. Paris: E. S. F.

Fabre, N. (1992). *Deux imaginaire pour une cure* [Two imaginaries for a cure]. Paris: Bayard Editeur.

Fabre, N. (1998). *Le travail de l'imaginaire en psychothérapie de l'enfant* [The work of the imaginary in child psychotherapy]. Paris: Dunod.

Fabre, N. (2002). *Allo specchio dei sogni* [Dreams in the mirror]. Roma: Magi.

Fabre, N. (2004). *L'immaginario in azione nella psicoterapia infantile* [The imaginary in action in child psychotherapy]. Roma: Magi.

Fabre, N. (2014, May). *Robert Desoille – Personal recollections.* Paper presented at the First International Conference on Waking Dream Therapy – Reveries from the past and stimuli to the future, Rabat, Malta.

Fabre, N., & Maurey, G. (1985). *Le rêve-éveillé analytique* [The analytic waking dream]. Toulouse: Privat.

Fabre, N., & Passerini, A. (2010). *Il rêve-éveillé dirigé in psicoterapia – via regia dell'immaginario* [The directed waking dream in psychotherapy – a royal road to the imaginary]. Roma: Alpes.

Favez-Boutonnier, J. (1945). *Contribution a la psychologie et la métaphysique de l'angoise* [A contribution towards a psychology and metaphysics of anguish]. Paris: Presses Universitaires de France.

Favez-Boutonnier, J. (1947). *L'angoisse* [Anguish]. These de doctorat des lettres, Université de Sorbonne, Paris.

Feld, A. (1990). Entretien avec Monique Tiberghien, onirotherapeute [Interview with Monique Tiberghien, oneirotherapist]. En N. Fabre & J. Launay (Eds.), *Hommage du centenaire – Robert Desoille*. Paris: Cahiers de'l'Institut Du Rêve-Éveillé En Psychoanalyse.

Ferro, A., & Civaterese, G. (2015). *The analytic field and its transformation*. London: Karnac Books.

Feurbach, L. (1862/1960). Das Geheimnis des Opfers oder der Mensch ist was er ißt [The secret of the victim or the man is what he eats]. In W. Bolin & F. Jodl (Eds.), *Ludwig Feuerbach Sämtliche Werke Bd.X* (pp. 41–67). Stuttgart-Bad Canstatt: Frommann Verlag.

Flournoy, T. (1963). *From India to the planet Mars*. New Hyde Park and New York: Univerisity Press. (Originally published in 1899).

Fonagy, P. (2001). *Attachment theory and psychoanalysis*. New York: Other Press.

Fordham, M. (1956). Active imagination and imaginative activity. *Journal of Analytical Psychology, 1*, 207–208.

Fordham, M. (1965). Des parents de bonne volonté ou l'importance du milieu dans la thérapie d'un enfant schizophrène [Parents of good will or the importance of the environment in a therapy of a schizophrenic child]. Action et Pensée, 1–2, Mars & Juin.

Fordham, M. (1967). Active imagination: De-integration or disintegration. *Journal of Analytical Psychology, 12*(1), 51–66.

Foucault, M. (1986a). Of other spaces (J. Miskowiec, Trans.). *Diacritics, 16*, Spring, 22. (Originally published as *Des espace autres* in 1967).

Foucault, M. (1986b). *The care of the self – The history of Sexuality*, Volume 3. London: Penguin Books.

Frank, L. (1910). *Die psychoanalyse* [Psychoanalysis]. Munich: E. Reinhardt.

Freud, S. (1950). Analysis, terminable and interminable. In J. Strachey (Ed. & Trans.), *The standard edition of the complete psychological works of Sigmund Freud*, Volume 5, (pp. 316–357). London: Hogarth Press. (Originally published 1937).

Freud, S. (1953a). Introductory lectures on Psycho-Analysis. In J. Strachey (Ed. & Trans.), *The standard edition of the complete psychological works of Sigmund Freud*, Volume 14, (pp. 241–463). London: Hogarth. (Originally published 1917).

Freud, S. (1953b). Three essays on the theory of sexuality. In J. Strachey (Ed. & Trans.), *The standard edition of the complete psychological works of Sigmund Freud*, Volume 7, (pp. 125–245). London: Hogarth Press. (Originally published in 1905).

Freud, S. (1957). On narcissism. In J. Strachey (Ed. & Trans.), *The standard edition of the complete psychological works of Sigmund Freud*, Volume 14, (pp. 67–102). London: Hogarth. (Originally published in 1914).

Freud, S. (1972). The relation of the poet to day-dreaming. In P. Rieff (Ed.), *Character and culture*. New York: Collier Books. (Originally published in 1908).

Freud, S., & Breuer, J. (1955). Studies on hysteria. In J. Strachey (Ed. & Trans.), *The standard edition of the complete psychological works of Sigmund Freud*, Volume 2, (pp. 19–305). London: Hogarth. (Originally published in 1895).

Furumoto, L. (1989). The new history of psychology. In I. S. Cohen (Ed.), *The G. Stanley Hall lecture series*, Volume 9, (pp. 9–34). Washington, DC: American Psychological Association.

Gabbard, G. (2004). *Long-term psychodynamic psychotherapy. A basic text.* Washington, DC: American Psychiatric Publishing.

Gaillard, C. (2012). The Egg, the vessels and the words. From Izdubar to answer to Job: For an imaging thinking (A. Conrade, Trans.). *Journal of Analytical Psychology, 57,* 299–334.

Gallard, M. (1994). Jung's attitude during the second World War in the light of the historical and professional context. *Journal of Analytical Psychology, 39,* 203–232.

Galton, F. (1881, May). The visions of sane persons. *Proceedings of the Royal Institution, 9,* 644–655.

Gantt, L., & Tinnin, L. (2009).Support for a neurobiological view of trauma with implications for art therapy. *The Arts in Psychotherapy, 36,* 148–153.

Gaudissart, I. (2014). *Love and sacrifice. The life of Emma Jung* (K. Llanwarne, Trans.). Asheville, NC: Chiron Publications.

Garfield, S., & Bergin, A. (1994). Introduction and historical overview. In A. Bergin & S. Garfield (Eds.), *Handbook of Psychotherapy and Behaviour Change,* (pp. 3–18). Chichester: Wiley.

Garufi, B. (1977). Reflections on the rêve éveillé dirigé method. *Journal of Analytical Psychology, 22*(3), 207–228.

Gaudé, S. (2006). Le cadre élaboré par la S.E.P.T. *Le Carnet PSY 2005/7* (n° 102), 24–25.

Gerard, R. (1961). The guided daydream in psychosynthesis. Fourteenth newsletter of Psychosynthesis Research Foundation, October, 1961. (Retrieved from: http://www.psychosynthesisresources.com/NieuweBestanden/NewslettersPRF.pdf)

Giegerich, W. (2007). *Technology and the soul: From the nuclear bomb to the world wide web.* New Orleans: Spring.

Giegerich, W. (2010). Liber Novus, that is, the New Bible, A first analysis of C. G. Jung's Red Book. *Spring, 83,* 361–413.

Gilbert, P. (2010). *Compassion-focused therapy: Distinctive features.* Hove: Routledge.

Gill, M. (1994). *Psychoanalysis in transition.* Hillsdale, NJ: Analytic Press.

Giovetti, P. (1995). *Roberto Assagioli: La vita e l'opera del fondatore della Psicosintesi* [Roberto Assagioli: The life and work of the founder of psychosynthesis]. Roma: Edizioni Mediterranee.

Gordon, R. (1968). Transference as a fulcrum of analysis. *Journal of Analytical Psychology, 13,* 109–117.

Gowan, J. C. (1975). *Trance, art, and creativity.* New York: Creative Education Foundation.

Greben, D. H. (2004). Integrative dimensions of psychotherapy training. *The Canadian Journal of Psychiatry, 49,* 238–248.

Greene, A. (2001). Conscious mind—conscious body. *Journal of Analytical Psychology, 46,* 565–590.

Griffin, D. R., Beardslee, W. A., & Holland, J. (1989). *Varieties of postmodern theology.* Albany: State University of New York Press.

Gross, F. L., & Gross, T. P. (1993). *The making of a mystic: Seasons in the life of Teresa of Avila.* Albany: State University of New York Press.

Groupe du rêve éveillé dirigé en psychothérapie (1967). Hommage a Monsieur Robert Desoille [A homage to Robert Desoille]. *Bulletin de la Societe de recherché psychotherapiques de langue francaise,* V,1, Mars, 1–38.

Guennon, R. (1971). *Études sur la Franc-Maçonnerie et le Compagnonnage* (Tome 1) [Studies on freemasonry]. Paris: Editions traditionelles.

Guerdon, D. (1993). *Le rêve éveillé, initiation pratique* [The waking dream, an initiatory practise]. Ile Saint-Denis: Oniros.

Guggisberg, M. (1995). Le psychothérapeute: Joseph Marc Narcisse Guillerey [The psychotherapist: Jospeh Marc Narcisse Guillerey]. In C. Muller (Ed.), *Portraits de psychiatres romands* (pp. 211–237). Nadir: Éditions Payot Lausanne.

Guillerey, M. (1945). Medicine psychologique [Psychological medecine]. In A. Carrel (Ed.), *Medecine officielle et medecins heretiques* (pp. 233–253). Paris: Plon.

Guillerey, M. (1955). Une nouvelle method psychothérapique [A new method of psychotherapy]. Conférence donnée en 1942. *Psyché, 10*(105), 405–436.

Guillhot, J. (1958). Second newsletter November, 1958 issued by the Psychosynthesis Research Foundation, Inc. U.S.A. (Retrieved from: http://www.psychosynthesisresources.com/NieuweBestanden/NewslettersPRF.pdf)

Guillhot, J. (2006, Fev). Rêve éveillé et psychosynthese [Waking dream and psychosynthesis]. *La Revue de Psychosynthese, 18*, 7–11.

Günther, M. (1990). The human voice: On Alfred Wolfsohn. *Spring, 50*, 65–75.

Hackmann, A., Bennett-Levy, J., & Holmes, E. A. (2011). *Oxford guide to imagery in cognitive therapy*. Oxford: Oxford University Press.

Hale, C. A. (2010). What about being red? Encounters with the color of Jung's Red Book. *Psychological Perspectives: A quarterly journal of Jungian thought, 53*(4), 479–494.

Haley, J. (1993). *Milton H. Erickson. A brief biography*. New York: Brunner/Mazel.

Hall, J. A. (1989). *Hypnosis: A Jungian perspective*. New York: Guilford Press.

Hall, J. A., & Brylowski, A. (1990). Lucid dreaming and active imagination: Implications for Jungian therapy. *Quadrant, 24*(1), 35–43.

Happich, C. (1932). Das Bildbewusstsein als ansatzstelle psychischer Behandlung [*Image consciousness as an addition to psychological treatment*]. *Zentralblatt fur psychotherapie, 5*, 633–643.

Hannah, B. (1953). Some remarks on active imagination. *Spring, 1953*, 38–58.

Hannah, B. (1981). *Encounters with the soul: Active imagination as developed by C. G. Jung*. Santa Monica: Sigo Press.

Hartmann, V. G. (1994). *The Franco-Prussian war or Jung as dissociationist*. Panel discussion on Psychological Authority at the October 26–30, 1994, conference of the Inter-Regional Society of Jungian Analysts at Asheville, North Carolina. (Retrieved from: http://www.cgjungpage.org/learn/articles/analytical-psychology/139-the-franco-prussian-war-or-jung-as-dissociationist)

Harris, M. J. (2008). *Folklore and the fantastic in 19th-century British fiction*. Aldershot: Ashgate.

Hauke, C. (2000). *Jung and the postmodern*. London: Routledge.

Hauke, C., & Alistair, I. (Eds.). (2001). *Jung and film: Post-Jungian takes on the moving image*. East Sussex: Brunner-Routledge.

Haule, J. R. (1984). From somnambulism to the archetypes: The French roots of Jung's split with Freud. *Psychoanalytic Review, 71*(4), 635–659.

Henderson, J. L. (1984). *Cultural attitudes in psychological perspective*. Toronto: Inner City Books.

Henriot, J. M. (2014, May). *Le transfert négatif en Psychanalyse Rêve Éveillé* [The negative transference in psychoanalytic waking dream]. Paper presented in the

First International Conference on Waking Dream Therapy – "Reveries from the past and stimuli to the future", Rabat, Malta.

Hillman, J. (1975). *Re-visioning psychology*. New York. Harper Colophon Books.

Hillman, J. (1979). *The dream and the underworld*. New York: Harper & Row.

Hillman, J. (1981). Psychology: Monotheistic or polytheistic. In D. L. Miller (Ed.), *The new polytheism: Rebrith of the gods and goddesses* (pp. 109–142). Dallas: Spring Publications.

Hillman, J. (1982). Anima mundi: The return of the soul to the world. *Spring*, 1982, 71–93.

Hillman, J. (1983). *Healing fiction*. New York: Station Hill Press.

Hillman, J. (1989). Imaginal practice: Greeting the angel. In T. Moore (Ed.), *Selected writings by James Hillman – A blue fire* (pp. 50–70). New York: Harper Perrenial.

Hillman, J. (1994). 'Man is by nature a political animal' or: Patient as citizen. In S. Shamdasani & M. Munchow (Eds.), *Speculations after Freud – Psychoanalysis, philosophy and culture* (pp. 29–40). London and New York: Routledge.

Hillman, J., & Pozzo, L. (1983). *Inter views: Conversations with Laura Pozzo on psychotherapy, biography, love, soul, dreams, work, imagination, and the state of the culture*. New York: Harper & Row.

Hillman, J., & Shamdasani, S. (2013). *Lament of the dead: Psychology after Jung's red book*. New York: W.W. Norton & Co.

Hillman, J., & Ventura, M. (1993). *We've had a hundred years of psychotherapy and the world is getting worse*. San Francisco: Harper.

Hockley, L. (2001). *Cinematic projections: The analytical psychology of C. G. Jung and film theory*. Luton: University of Luton Press.

Hockley, L. (2007). *Frames of mind: A post-Jungian look at cinema, television and technology*. Bristol: Intellect Books.

Hoffman, I. Z. (1998). *Ritual and spontaneity in the psychoanalytic process. A dialectical-constructivist view*. Hillsdale, NJ: Analytic Press.

Holmes, J. (1993). *John Bowlby and attachment theory*. London: Routledge.

Holmes, J. (2014). *The Therapeutic imagination: Using literature to deepen psychodynamic understanding and enhance empathy*. New York: Routledge.

Horowitz, M. J., & Becker, S. (1971). Cognitive response to stressful stimuli. *Archives of General Psychiatry, 25*, 419–428.

Humbert, E. (1971a). Active imagination: Theory and practice. *Spring*, 1971, 101–114.

Humbert, E. (1971b, Nov–Dec). L'imagination active [Active imagination]. *Psychotherapies: Revue de l'Arbre Vert, 3*, 11–12.

Humbert, E. (1979). Il ruolo dell'immagine nella psicologia analitica [The role of the image in analytical psychology]. *Rivista di Psicologia Analitica, 20*, 31–64.

Humbert, E. (1980). Active imagination: Questioned and discussed. In I. F. Baker (Ed.), *Methods of treatment in analytical psychology – V11 International congress of the international association for analytical psychology* (pp. 134–138). Fellbach: Bonz.

Izod, J. (2000). Active imagination and the analysis of film. *Journal of Analytical Psychology, 45*(2), 267–285.

Jackson, R. (1981). *Fantasy: The literature of subversion*. London: Routledge.

Jackson, E. (1996). *Food and transformation. Imagery and symbolism of eating.* Toronto: Inner City Books.

James, W. (1985). *The varieties of religious experience.* New York: Penguin Classics. (Originally published in 1902).

James, W. (1906). *L'experience religieuse. Essai de psycholgie descriptive* [The religious experience. An essay on descriptive psychology]. (F. Abauzit Trans.). Paris: Alcan and Geneve: Kundig.

James, W. (1907). The energies of men. *Science*, N.S. *25*(635), 321–332.

James, W. (1911). *On vital reserves: The energies of men.* New York: H. Holt.

James, W. (1920). *The letters of William James – In two volumes*, Henri James (Ed.). Boston: The Atlantic Monthly Press.

Jameson, F. (1991). *Postmodernism or the cultural logic of late capitalism.* Durham, NC: Duke University Press.

Janet, P. (1898). *Névroses et idées fixes* [Neurosis and fixed ideas]. Paris: Alcan.

Janet, P. (1927). *De l'angoise a l'extase* [From anguish to ecstasy]. Paris: Alcan.

Jenny, L. (1997). *L'experience de la chute de Montaigne a Michaux.* [The experience of the fall from Montainge to Michaux]. Paris: Presse Universitaires de France.

Jensen, J. P., Bergin, A., & Greaves, D. W. (1990). The meaning of eclecticism: New survey and analysis of components. *Professional Psychology, 21*, 124–130.

Johnson, R. (1986). *Inner work: Using dreams and active imagination for personal growth.* New York: Harper Collins.

Jones, D, Vinton, M., & Wernick, W. (1999, November 21). *Three perspectives: Framing the Don Jones Assessment (DJS).* Panel presentation, American Art Therapy Association conference, Orlando, FL.

Jung. C. G. (1926). *Métamorphoses et symboles de la libido* [Metamorphosis and symbols of the libido]. Paris: Montaigne.

Jung, C. G. (1928a, Nov–Dec). La structure de l'âme [The structure of the soul]. *Revue Metapsychique, 6*, 472–490.

Jung, C. G. (1928b). *L'inconscient dans la vie psychique normale et abnormale* [The unconscious in the normal and abnormal psychic life] (Dr Grandjean-Bayard, Trans.). Paris: Payot.

Jung, C. G. (1931a). *Essais de psychologie analytique* (Y. Le Lay, Trans.) [Essays on analytical psychology]. Paris: Delamain et Boutelleau.

Jung, C. G. (1931b). Psychological types. *Action et Pensée, 1*, Jan, 18–23.

Jung, C. G. (1931c). Psychological types. *Action et Pensée, 2*, Fev, 54–68.

Jung, C. G. (1931d). Psychological types. *Action et Pensée, 3*, Mars, 106–115.

Jung. C. G. (1933). Seelenprobleme der Gegenwart [The problems of modern soul]. *Action et Pensée, 4*, Avril.

Jung. C. G. (1938a). *Le Moi e l'Inconscient* [The ego and the unconscious]. Paris: Gallimard.

Jung. C. G. (1938b). *Phenomenes occultes* [Occult phenomena]. Paris: Montaigne.

Jung, C. G. (1938–1939). *Notes on Lectures given at the Eidgenossische Technische Hochschule, Zurich by Prof. C. G. Jung between 1938–1939.* ETH lectures recorded by Barbara Hannah. Unpublished manuscript.

Jung, C. G. (1939–1940). *Exercitia Spiritualia of St. Ignatius of Loyola. Notes on Lectures given at the Eidgenossische Technische Hochschule, Zurich by*

Prof. C. G. Jung between June 1939–May 1940. ETH lectures recorded by Barbara Hannah. Unpublished manuscript.

Jung, C. G. (1944, Fev). L'expérience des associations [The experience of associations]. *Action et Pensée,* . 1, 1–11.

Jung, C. G. (1960). Spirit and life. In H. Read, M. Fordham, G. Adler, & W. McGuire (Eds.), *Collected works volume 8: The structure and the dynamics of the psyche.* (R. F. C. Hull. Trans.). (pp. 319–337). Princeton, NJ: Princeton University Press. (Originally published in 1926).

Jung, C. G. (1960a). On psychic energy. In H. Read, M. Fordham, G. Adler, & W. McGuire (Eds.). *Collected works volume 8: The structure and the dynamics of the psyche.* (R. F. C. Hull. Trans.). (pp. 3–66). Princeton, NJ: Princeton University Press. (Originally published in 1948).

Jung, C. G. (1960b). The transcendent function. In H. Read, M. Fordham, G. Adler, & W. McGuire (Eds.), *Collected works volume 8: The structure and the dynamics of the psyche.* (R. F. C. Hull. Trans.). (pp. 67–91). New York: Bollingen Foundation. (Originally published in 1916).

Jung, C. G. (1961a). The theory of psychoanalysis. In W. McGuire (Exec. Ed.), Sir H. Read, M. Fordham, & G. Adler (Eds.). *Collected works volume 4: Freud and psychoanalysis,* (R. F. C. Hull. Trans.). (pp. 85–228). Princeton, NJ: Princeton University Press. (Originally published in 1913).

Jung, C. G. (1961b). Some crucial points in psychoanalysis: A correspondence between Dr. Jung and Dr. Loy. In W. McGuire (Exec. Ed.), Sir H. Read, M. Fordham, & G. Adler (Eds.). *Collected works volume 4: Freud and psychoanalysis.* (R. F. C. Hull. Trans.). (pp. 252–289). Princeton, NJ: Princeton University Press. (Originally published in 1914).

Jung, C. G. (1966a). The structure of the unconscious. In W. McGuire (Exec. Ed.), Sir H. Read, M. Fordham, & G. Adler (Eds.). *Collected works volume 7: Two essays on analytical psychology.* (R. F. C. Hull, Trans.). (pp. 269–304). Princeton, NJ: Princeton University Press. (Originally published in 1916).

Jung. C. G. (1966b). The technique of differentiation between the ego and the figures of the unconscious. In W. McGuire (Exec. Ed.), Sir H. Read, M. Fordham, & G. Adler (Eds.). *Collected works volume 7: Two essays on analytical psychology.* (R. F. C. Hull. Trans.). (pp. 212–226). Princeton, NJ: Princeton University Press. (Originally published in 1928).

Jung. C. G. (1966c). The aims of psychotherapy. In W. McGuire (Exec. Ed.), Sir H. Read, M. Fordham, & G. Adler (Eds.). *Collected works volume 16: The practice of psychotherapy.* (R. F. C. Hull, Trans.). (pp. 36–52). Princeton, NJ: Princeton University Press. (Originally published in 1931).

Jung, C. G. (1966d). Appendix: The realities of practical psychotherapy. In W. McGuire (Exec. Ed.), Sir H. Read, M. Fordham, & G. Adler (Eds.). *Collected works volume 16: The practice of psychotherapy* (R. F. C. Hull, Trans.). (pp. 327–338). Princeton, NJ: Princeton University Press. (Originally published in 1937).

Jung, C. G. (1966e). The psychology of the transference. In H. Read, M. Fordham, G. Adler, & W. McGuire (Eds.). *Collected works volume. 16: The practice of psychotherapy.* (R. F. C. Hull. Trans.). (pp. 164–323). Princeton, NJ: Princeton University Press. (Originally published in 1946).

Jung, C. G. (1966f). Problems of modern psychotherapy. In H. Read, M. Fordham, G. Adler, & W. McGuire (Eds.). *Collected works volume. 16: The practice of psychotherapy.* (R. F. C. Hull. Trans.). (pp. 53–75). Princeton, NJ: Princeton University Press. (Originally published in 1931).

Jung, C. G. (1966g). *Collected works volume 15: The spirit in man, art and literature.* (W. McGuire [Exec. Ed.], Sir H. Read, M. Fordham, G. Adler [Eds.] & R. F. C. Hull. [Trans.]). Princeton, NJ: Princeton University Press.

Jung, C. G. (1967a). *Collected works volume 5: Symbols of Transformation.* (W. McGuire [Exec. Ed.], Sir H. Read, M. Fordham, G. Adler [Eds.] & R. F. C. Hull. [Trans.]). Princeton, NJ: Princeton University Press. (Originally published in 1912).

Jung, C. G. (1967b). Commentary on "The secret of the golden flower". In W. McGuire (Exec. Ed.), Sir H. Read, M. Fordham, & G. Adler (Eds.). *Collected works volume 13: Alchemical studies.* (R. F. C. Hull, Trans.). (pp. 1–54). Princeton, NJ: Princeton University Press. (Originally published in 1929).

Jung, C. G. (1967c). The philosophical tree. In W. McGuire (Exec. Ed.), Sir H. Read, M. Fordham, & G. Adler (Eds.). *Collected works volume 13: Alchemical studies.* (R. F. C. Hull, Trans.). (pp. 251–349). Princeton, NJ: Princeton University Press. (Originally published in 1954).

Jung, C. G. (1967d). *C. G. Jung bibliothek, katalog.* [C. G. Jung's library, catalogue]. Kusnacht – Zurich.

Jung. C. G. (1968a). A study in the process of individuation. In W. McGuire (Exec. Ed.), Sir H. Read, M. Fordham, & G. Adler (Eds.). *Collected works volume 9: The archetypes and the collective unconscious.* (R. F. C. Hull, Trans.). (pp. 290–354). Princeton, NJ: Princeton University Press. (Originally published in 1933).

Jung, C. G. (1968b). Psychological aspects of the mother archetype. In W. McGuire (Exec. Ed.), Sir H. Read, M. Fordham, & G. Adler (Eds.). *Collected works volume 9i: The archetypes and the collective unconscious.* (R. F. C. Hull, Trans.). (pp. 75–110). Princeton, NJ: Princeton University Press. (Originally published in 1941).

Jung, C. G. (1968c). On the psychology of the trickster-figure. In W. McGuire (Exec. Ed.), Sir H. Read, M. Fordham, & G. Adler (Eds.). *Collected works volume 9i: The archetypes and the collective unconscious.* (R. F. C. Hull, Trans.). (pp. 255–272). Princeton, NJ: Princeton University Press. (Originally published in 1954).

Jung, C. G. (1968d). Appendix: Mandalas. In W. McGuire (Exec. Ed.), Sir H. Read, M. Fordham, & G. Adler (Eds.). *Collected works volume 9i: The archetypes and the collective unconscious.* (R. F. C. Hull, Trans.). (pp. 385–390). Princeton, NJ: Princeton University Press. (Originally published in 1955).

Jung, C. G. (1968e). *Collected works volume 12: Psychology and alchemy.* (W. McGuire [Exec. Ed.], Sir H. Read, M. Fordham, G. Adler [Eds.] & R. F. C. Hull. [Trans.]). Princeton, NJ: Princeton University Press. (Originally published in 1944).

Jung. C. G. (1968f). The phenomenology of the spirit in fairytales. In W. McGuire (Exec. Ed.), Sir H. Read, M. Fordham, & G. Adler (Eds.). *Collected works volume 9i: The archetypes and the collective unconscious.* (R. F. C. Hull, Trans.). (pp. 207–254). Princeton, NJ: Princeton University Press. (Originally published in 1948).

Jung. C. G. (1969a). Psychological commentary on the "Tibetan book of great liberation". In W. McGuire (Exec. Ed.), Sir H. Read, M. Fordham, & G. Adler

(Eds.). *Collected works volume11: Psychology and religion: West and east.* (R. F. C. Hull, Trans.). (pp. 494–508) Princeton, NJ: Princeton University Press. (Originally published in 1939).

Jung, C. G. (1969b). Answer to Job. In W. McGuire (Exec. Ed.), Sir H. Read, M. Fordham, & G. Adler (Eds.). *Collected works volume 11: Psychology and religion: West and east.* (R. F. C. Hull, Trans.). (pp. 355–470). Princeton, NJ: Princeton University Press. (Originally published in 1954).

Jung. C. G. (1969c). Yoga and the west. In W. McGuire (Exec. Ed.), Sir H. Read, M. Fordham, & G. Adler (Eds.). *Collected volume 11: Psychology and religion: West and East.* (R. F. C. Hull. Trans.). (pp. 529–537). Princeton, NJ: Princeton University Press. (Originally published in 1936).

Jung, C. G. (1969d). *Collected works volume 9ii: Aion – Researches into the phenemonology of the self.* (W. McGuire [Exec. Ed.], Sir H. Read, M. Fordham, G. Adler [Eds.] & R. F. C. Hull. [Trans.]). Princeton, NJ: Princeton University Press.

Jung, C. G. (1970a). *Collected works volume 14: Mysterium coniunctionis.* (W. McGuire [Exec. Ed.], Sir H. Read, M. Fordham, G. Adler [Eds.] & R. F. C. Hull. [Trans.]). Princeton, NJ: Princeton University Press. (Originally published in 1955).

Jung, C. G. (1970b). On the psychology and pathology of so-called occult phenomena. In W. McGuire (Exec. Ed.), Sir H. Read, M. Fordham, & G. Adler (Eds.). *Collected works volume 1: Psychiatric Studies* (R. F. C. Hull. Trans.). (pp. 3–92). Princeton, NJ: Princeton University Press. (Originally published in 1902).

Jung. C. G. (1971). *Collected works volume 6: Psychological Types.* (W. McGuire [Exec. Ed.], Sir H. Read, M. Fordham, G. Adler [Eds.] & R. F. C. Hull. [Trans.]). Princeton, NJ: Princeton University Press. (Originally published in 1921).

Jung, C. G. (1973). *Letters, vol, 1 (1906–1950).* Princeton, NJ: Princeton University Press.

Jung, C. G. (1975). *Letters, vol, 2 (1951–1961).* Princeton, NJ: Princeton University Press.

Jung, C. G. (1976a). The Tavistock lectures: On the theory and practisce of analytical psychology. In W. McGuire (Exec. Ed.), Sir H. Read, M. Fordham, & G. Adler (Eds.). *Collected works volume 18: The symbolic life.* (R. F. C. Hull, Trans.). (pp. 5–182). Princeton, NJ: Princeton University Press. (Originally published in 1935).

Jung, C. G. (1976b). Foreword to von Koenig-Fachsenfeld: Wandlungen des Traumproblmes von der Romatik bis zur Gegenwart. In W. McGuire (Exec. Ed.), Sir H. Read, M. Fordham, & G. Adler (Eds.). *Collected works volume 18: The symbolic life.* (R. F. C. Hull, Trans.). (pp. 5–182). Princeton, NJ: Princeton University Press. (Originally published in 1935).

Jung, C. G. (1984). *Dream Analysis: Notes on the seminar given in (1928–1930).* W. McGuire (Ed.). Princeton, NJ: Princeton University Press.

Jung. C. G. (1989). *Analytical psychology: Notes on the seminar given in 1925.* W. McGuire, (Ed.). Princeton, NJ: Princeton University Press. (Originally published in 1925).

Jung, C. G. (1995). *Memories, dreams, reflections.* London: Fontana Press. (Originally published in 1963).

Jung. C. G. (1996). *The psychology of Kundalini yoga. Notes on the seminar given in 1932.* S. Shamdasani (Ed.). Princeton, NJ: Princeton University Press.

Jung, C. G. (1998a). *Visions. Notes of the seminar given in 1930–1934.* Volume 1. C. Douglas (Ed.). London: Routledge.

Jung, C. G. (1998b). *Visions. Notes of the seminar given in 1930–1934.* Volume 2. C. Douglas (Ed.). London: Routledge.

Jung, C. G. (2009). *The Red Book, Liber Novus.* (Ed. Sonu Shamdasani. Trans. Mark Kyburz, John Peck, & Sonu Shamdasani). New York: W.W Norton & Company.

Jung, C. G. (2014). *Nietzche's Zarathustra: Notes of the seminar given in 1934–39. Vol 2.* J. L. Jarrett (Ed.). East Sussex: Routledge.

Jung, E. (1957). The anima as an elemental being. In *Anima and animus: Two essays* (pp. 45–87). New York: The Analytical Psychology Club.

Kalff, D. (1980). *Sandplay, a psychotherapeutic approach to the psyche.* Santa Monica, CA: Sigo Press.

Kast, V. (1988). *Imagination as a space of freedom: Dialogue between the ego and the unconscious.* New York: International Publishing Corp.

Kast, V. (1993). *Through emotions to maturity. Psychological readings of fairy-tales.* New York: Fromm International Pub Corp.

Kast, V. (2014). Complexes and imagination. *Journal of Analytical Psychology, 59*(5), 680–694.

Kaufmann, Y. (2009). *The way of the image. The orientational approach to the psyche.* New York: Zahav Books.

Keller, T. (1940). *L'ame et le nerfs* (PP/TKR/7) [The soul and nerves]. Tina Keller Papers, Archives of the Wellcome Library, London.

Keller, T (1941). L'imagination active [Active imagination]. *Action et Pensée, 3,* Sept, 76–83.

Keller, A. (1955). C. G. Jung et la crise de notre temps [C. G. Jung and the crisis of our times]. *Action et Pensée, 3,* Sept., 65–72.

Keller, T. (1979). *Recollections of my encounter with Dr. Jung.* Tina Keller Papers, Archives of the Wellcome Library, London.

Keller, T. (1981). *Autobiography* (Unpublished manuscript in English). Keller Family Papers, Geneva, Switzerland.

Kemp, R. (1950, Oct). La psychologie de Jung [The psychology of Jung]. *Nouvelles Litteraires, 19.*

Kernberg, O. F. (1993). Convergences and divergences in contemporary psychoanalytic technique. *The International Journal of Psychoanalysis, 74,* 659–673.

Keutzer, C. S. (1984). Synchronicity in psychotherapy. *Journal of Analytical Psychology, 29,* 373–381.

Keyserling, H. (1938). *From suffering to fulfillment.* Plymouth: Brandon & Son.

Khan, M. R. (1986). Holding and interpretation. *International Psycho-Analytic Library, 115,* 1–194. London: The Hogarth Press and the Institute of Psycho-Analysis.

Kirsch, T. (2000). *The Jungians: A comparative and historical perspective.* London: Routledge.

Kirsch, T., & Hogenson, G. (Eds.). (2014). *The red book. Reflections on C. G. Jung's liber novus.* London & New York: Routledge.

Kittleson, M. L. (1996). *Sounding the soul: Listening to the psyche.* Einsiedeln, Switzerland: Daimon.

Klein, M. (1928). Early stages of the Oedipus conflict. *International Journal of Psycho-Analysis, 9*, 167–180.

Kluft, R. P. (1989). Playing for time: Temporizing techniques in the treatment of multiple personality disorder. *American Journal of Clinical Hypnosis, 32*(2), 90–98.

Kluge, H., & Thren, H. (1951). Bildstreifendenken als psychotherapeutische methode [Thinking as in a movie as a form of psychotherapy]. *Zentralblatt fur psychotherapie, 1*, 13–19.

Kosslyn, S. M., Ganis, G., & Thompson, W. L. (2009). Mental imagery. In G. G. Bernston, & J. T. Cacioppo, (Eds.), *Handbook of neuroscience for the behavioral sciences*, Volume 1, (pp. 383–339). New York: Wiley & Sons.

Kovacev, A. N. (2009). The return to the origins: Jung, Wagner and symbolic forms. *Musicological Annual, XLV*(1), 89–115.

Kraidy, M. M. (2005). *Hybridity, or the cultural logic of globalisation*. Philadelphia: Temple University Press.

Kramer, E. (2000). The art therapist's third hand. In L. A. Gerity (Ed.), *Art as therapy – Collected papers by Edith Kramer* (pp. 47–70). London and Philadelphia: Jessica Kingsley Publishers.

Kretschmer, E. (1952). *A Text-book of medical psychology*. London: Hogarth. (Originally published in 1922).

Kretschmer, W. (1966). Meditative techniques in psychotherapy. In C. Tart (Ed.), *Altered states of consciousness* (pp. 224–233). New York: John Wiley.

Kroke, A. (2004). L'usa dell'immaginazione attiva nella seduta analitica: alcuni aspetti terapeutici [The use of active imagination in the analytic session: Certain therapeutic aspects]. *Studi Junghiani, 20* (Luglio/Dicembre).

Kroke, A. (2013). Brevi indicazione teorico-pratiche sull'immaginazione attiva [Brief theoretical-practical indications on active imagination]. *Quaderni di Cultura Junghiana, Anno 2, numero, 2*, 74–76.

Kunzendorf, R. G., & Sheikh, A. (1990). *The psychophysiology of mental imagery: Theory, research and application*. Amityville, NY: Baywood.

Lachapelle, S. (2011). *Investigating the supernatural. From spritism and occultism to psychical research and metaphysics in France, 1853–1931*. Baltimore: The John Hopkins University Press.

Lakoff, G., & Johnson, M. (1980). *Metaphors we live by*. Chicago, IL: University of Chicago Press.

Lampropoulos, G. K. (2001). Bridging technical eclecticism and theoretical integration: Assimilative integration. *Journal of Psychotherapy Integration, 11*, 5–19.

Lang, P. J., Greenwald, M. K., Bradley, & M. M., Hamm, A. O. (1993). Looking at pictures: Affective, facial, visceral, and behavioral reactions. *Psychophysiology, 20*, 261–273.

Laplanche, J., & Pontalis, J. B. (1973). *The language of psycho-analysis* (D. Nicholson-Smith, Trans.). New York: W. W. Norton.

Lapworth, P., & Sills, C. (2010). *Integration in counselling and psychotherapy*, 2nd ed. London, Thousand Oaks and New Delhi: Sage.

Larsen, S. (1996). *The mythic imagination. The quest for meaning through personal mythology*. Vermont: Inner traditions.

Latour, B. (1970, August 24). *Carl Gustav Jung ou la totalite de l'homme future: Symbole dus soi et individuation. 3rd series on Jung* - Radio programme with the participation of E. Humbert, M. V. Franz, J. Jacobi, G. Durand, A. Virel. (Retreived from: http://www.ina.fr/audio/PHD99213327).

Launay, J., Levine, J., & Maurey, G. (1975). *Le rêve éveillé dirigé et l'inconscient* [The directed waking dream and the unconscious]. Bruxelles: Dessart et Mardaga

Launay, J. (1983). Le rêve éveillé et l'inconscient [The waking dream and the unconscious]. In Y. Pelicier (Dir.), *La serrure et le songe. L'activite mental du sommeil* (pp. 181–194). Paris: Economica.

Lawrence, W. G. (2003). *Experiences in social dreaming*. London: Karnac Books.

Lebois, A. (1955). Réflexions sur les archétypes [Reflections on the archetypes]. *Le Disque Vert*, Bruxelles, 205–219.

Lecchi, P. (2015). Esperienza immaginativa in pedagogia: Il laboratorio delle emozioni [Imaginative experience in pedagogy: The laboratory of emotions]. In A. Passerini & F. Vegetti (eds), *Esperienza Immaginativa: Counseling, pedagogia e psicoterapia* [Imaginative experience: Counseling, pedagogy and psychotherapy] (pp. 95–142). Rome: Alpes.

Lefebvre, H. (1991). *The production of space* (D. Nicholson-Smith, Trans.). Oxford: Blackwell.

Leuba, H. J. (1925). *Psychologie du mysticisme religieux* (L. Herr, Trad.) [The psychology of religious mysticism]. Paris: Alcan.

Leuner, H. (1969). Guided affective imagery (GAI). A method of intensive psychotherapy. *American Journal of Psychotherapy*, 23(1), 4–21.

Levebre, H. (1976). Reflections on the politics of space. *Antipode*, 8, 30–37.

Levi-Strauss, C. (1964). *Mythologiques, t. I: Le Cru et le Cuit* [Mythological: The raw and the cooked]. Paris: Plon.

Lewis, P. (1982). Authentic movement as active imagination. In J. Hariman (Ed.) *The compendium of psychotherapeutic techniques* (pp. 75–100). Springfield, IL: Charles C. Thomas, Publisher.

Lijphart, A. (1971, Sept). Comparative politics and the comparative method. *American Political Science Review*, 65, 682–693.

Liljefors, N. (2009). Le rêve éveillé en psychotherapie courte. Quelques experiences [The waking dream in brief psychotherapy. Some experiences]. *Imaginaire et Inconscient*, 23, 97–114.

Loewenthal, D., & Samuels, A. (Eds.) (2014). *Relational psychoanalysis, psychotherapy and counselling*. London: Routledge.

Lopez-Pedraza, R. (1977). *Hermes and his children*. Zurich: Spring Publications.

Lorenzo, D. S. (1970). Il metodo dell'immaginazione attiva nella psicologia di C. G. Jung [The method of active imagination in the psychology of C. G. Jung]. *Rivista di Psicologia Analitica*, 2, 305–386.

Lowen, A. (1975). *Bioenergetics*. New York: Penguin Books.

Lu, K. (2011). Jung and history. In G. Heuer (Ed.), *Sexual revolutions* (pp. 11–34). London: Routledge.

Lu, K. (2012). Jung history and his approach to the psyche. *Journal of Jungian Scholarly Studies*, 8(9), 1–24.

Lubac, H., Rougier, M., & Sales, M. (1985). *Gabriel Marcel – Gaston Fessard, Correspondence (1934–1971)*. Paris: Beauchesne.

Luborsky, L., & Crits-Christoph, P. (1990). *Understanding transference: The CCRT method*. New York: Basic Books.

Lusebrink, V. (1990). *Imagery and visual expression in therapy*. New York: Plenum Press.

Machtiger, H. G. (1984). Reflections on the transference/countertransference process with borderline patients. In N. Schwartz-Salant & M. Stein (Eds.), *Transference/countertransference: The Chiron clinical series* (pp. 119–145).Wilmette, IL: Chiron Publications.

Machtiger, H. G. (1995). Countertransference. In M. Stein (Ed.), *Jungian analysis* (2nd ed., pp. 210–237). Chicago, IL: Open Court.

Maguire, W. M. (2006). *The conversion of imagination. From Pascal to Rousseau to Tocqueville*. Cambridge, MA: Harvard University Press.

Maidi, H. (1983). *Rorschach et rêve éveillé dirigé dans l'etude de la personalite adolescente – contribution de l'analyse phenomeno-structurale* [Rorschach and directed waking dream in the study of a personality of an adolescent – an analytic contribution of the phenomenal-structural]. These de psychologie, Université de Lille III.

Malan, B. (1975). *Contribution a l'etude historique du rêve éveillé dirigé en psychothérapie* [A contribution of the historical study of directed waking dream in psychotherapy]. These Pour le doctorat en medicin, Faculté Mixte de Médecine et de Pharmacie de Rouen.

Malinowski, B. (1954). *Magic, science and religion*. New York: Anchor Books.

Marcel. G. (1938). Exploration de l'affectivité subconsciente par la méthode du rêve éveillé [An exploration of sub-conscious emotions in the waking dream method]. *Revue La Vie Intellectuelle, LV11*, 417–418.

Marcel, G. (1951). *The mystery of being. Vol. 1.* (G. S. Fraser, Trans.). London: The Harvill Press.

Marechal, J. (1924). *Etudes sur la psycholgie des mystiques* [Studies on the psychology of mystics]. Paris: Alcan.

Marjula, A. (1967). The healing influence of active imagination in a specific case of neurosis. In B. Hannah (Ed.), *Encounters with the soul: Active imagination as developed by C. G. Jung* (pp. 133–218). Santa Monica: Sigo Press.

Martin-Vallas, F. (2013). Une préface à 'La structure de l'âme' de C. G. Jung [A preface to the "Structure of the soul"]. *Revue de Psychologie Analytique, 1*, 163–176.

Marwick, A. (2001). *The new nature of history*. Basingstoke, Hampshire: Palgrave Macmillan.

Massey, D. (1994). *Space, place, and gender*. Minneapolis: University of Minnesota Press.

Massey, D. (1995). *Spatial divisions of labor: Social structures and the geography of production*. New York: Routledge.

Massey, D. (2005). *For space*. London: Sage.

Mauco, G. (1953). Le rêve éveillé dans le traitement psychoanalytique de l'enfant [The waking dream in the psychoanalytic treatment of a child]. *Action et Pensee, 29*, 2–3.

Maurey, G. (1995). *Le rêve-éveillé en psychoanalyse. De l'imaginaire a l'inconscient* [The waking dream in psychoanalysis. From the imaginary to the unconscious]. Paris: ESF.

Mauz, F. (1948). Der psychotische mensch in der psychotherapie [The psychotic person in psychotherapy]. *Arch Psychiatr Nervenk, 181*, 337–341.

McGuire, W. (Ed.). (1974). *The Freud/Jung letters: The correspondence between Sigmund Freud and C. G. Jung.* London: The Hogarth Press and Routledge & Kegan Paul.

McGuire, W., & Hull, R. F. C. (1977). *C. G. Jung speaking – Interviews and encounters.* Princeton, NJ: Princeton University Press.

McLynn, F. (1996). *Carl Gustav Jung.* New York: St. Martin's Press.

McNamee, S. (2002). The social construction of disorders: From pathology to potential. In J. D. Raskin & S. K. Bridges (Eds.), *Studies in meaning: Exploring constructivist psychology.* New York: Pace University Press.

McNamee, S., & Gergen, K. J. (1999). *Relational responsibility: Resources for sustainable dialogue.* Thousand Oaks, CA: Sage, Inc.

McNeely, D. (1987). *Touching: Body therapy and depth psychology.* Toronto: Inner City Books.

McWilliams, N. (1994). *Psychoanalytic diagnosis: Understanding personality structure in the clinical process.* New York: Guilford Press.

Meier, C. A. (2009). *Healing dream and ritual.* Einsiedeln, Switzerland: Daimon Verlag. (Originally published in 1949).

Merkur, D. (1993). *Gnosis: An esoteric tradition of mystical visions and unions.* Albany: State University of New York Press.

Merleau-Ponty, M. (1962). *Phenomenology of perception,* C. Smith (Trans.). London: Routledge.

Messer, S. B. (2001). Introduction to special on assimilative integration. *Journal of Psychotherapy Integration, 11*(1), 1–4.

Meyer, R. (2007). *Clio's circle: Entering the imaginal world of historians.* New Orleans: Spring Journal Books.

Miller, J. C. (2004). *The transcendent function.* Albany: State University of New York Press.

Milner, M. (1950). *On not being able to paint.* Madisson, CT: International Universities Press.

Mindell, A. (1985). *Working with the dreaming body.* London: Arkana.

Mitchell, S. A. (1988). *Relational concepts in psychoanalysis.* Cambridge, MA: Harvard University Press.

Mitchell, S. A. (2000). *Relationality: From attachment to intersubjectivity.* Mahwah, NJ: Analytic Press.

Mitchell, S. A., & Aron, L. (Eds.). (1999). *Relational psychoanalysis: The emergence of a tradition.* Hillsdale, NJ: The Analytic Press.

Mogenson, G. (1992). Living the symptom. *The Psychotherapy Patient, 8*(3/4), 11–25.

Montoro, L., Tortosa, F., Carpintero, H., & Peiro, J. M. (1984). A short history of the International Congresses of Psychology (1889–1960). *Revista de Historia de la Psicología, 5,* 245–253.

Moore, R. L., & Gillette, D. (1991). *King, warrior, magician, lover: Rediscovering the archetypes of the mature masculine.* San Francisco: Harper

Morgan, R., & Bakan, P. (1965). Sensory deprivation hallucinations and other sleep behaviour as a function of postion, method of report and anxiety. *Perceptual and Motor Skills, 20,* 19–25.

Nachmansohn, N. (1957). Concerning experimentally produced dreams. In D. Rapaport (Ed.), *The organisation and pathology of thought* (pp. 257–287). New York: Columbia University Press.

Nadal, J. (1967). Psychothérapie d'enfant par le R.E.D. [Child psychotherapy with R.E.D.]. *Bulletin de la Société de Recherché Psychothérapiques de Langue Francaise*, 5(1), 35–38.

Nadal, J. (1969). Approche de l'imaginaire chez l'enfant par le R.E.D. [An imaginary approach with children through R.E.D.]. *Bulletin de la Société de Recherché Psychotéhrapiques de Langue Francaise*, 7(1), 25–27.

Negley, S. C. (2014). The coniunctio gastronomique: Reflections on the process of individuation in culinary terms. *Psychological Perspectives*, 57(4), 384–402.

Neimeyer, R. A., (2000). Narrative disruptions in the construction of the self. In R. A. Neimeyer and J. D. Raskin (Eds.), *Constructions of disorder: Meaning-making frameworks for psychotherapy* (pp. 207–242). Washington, DC: American Psychological Association.

Newham, P. (1993). *The singing cure: An introduction to voice movement therapy.* London; Rider & Co.

Nora, P. (1984). *Les lieux des memoires.* [Places of memory]. Paris: Gallimard.

Norcross, J., & Goldfried, M. R. (2005). *Handbook of psychotherapy integration* (2nd edition). New York: Oxford University Press.

Nucho, O. Aina. (2003). *The psychoocybernetic model of art therapy.* Springfield, IL: Charles C. Thomas Pub. Ltd.

Ogden, T. H. (1994). *Subjects of analysis.* Northvale, NJ: Jason Aronson.

Ogden, T. (2005). On psychoanalytic supervision. *International Journal of Psychoanalysis*, 86(5), 1265–1280.

O'Hara, D., & Schofield, M. (2008). Personal approaches to psychotherapy integration. *Counselling and Psychotherapy Research*, 8(1), 53–62.

Oldmeadow, H. (1995). *Mircea Eliade & Carl Jung: Priests without surplices?* Department of Arts, La Trobe University Bendigo, (Studies in western traditions: Occasional papers, 1).

Øyen, E. (Ed.) (1990). *Comparative methodology: Theory and practice in international social research.* London: Sage.

Paige, N. (2000). *Being interior: Autobiography and the contradictions of modernity in seventeenth century France.* Philadelphia: University of Pennsylvania Press.

Pallaro, P. (1999). *Authentic movement: Essays by Mary Starks Whitehouse, Janet Adler, and Joan Chodorow.* Philadelphia: Jessica Kingsley Publishers.

Papasogli. B. (1991). *Il "fondo del cuore". Figure dello spazio interiore nel Seicento francese* ["The bottom of the heart". Figures of interior space in sixteenth century France]. Pisa: Goliardica.

Pardo, E. *Pantheatre.* (Retreived from: http://www.pantheatre.com/)

Passerini, A. (2009). *Immaginario: Cura e creativita'* [Imaginary: Cure and creativity]. Roma: Alpes.

Passerini, A. (2011). Il potere curativo dell'esperienza immaginativa nella psicoterapia sessuale. *Sessuologia*, 2(35), 115–120.

Passerini, A., & Toller, G. (2007). *Psicoterapia con la procedura immaginativa – metapsicologia e cenni metodologici* [Psychotherapy with imaginative procedure: Methodological and metapsychological aspects]. Roma: Armando.

Passerini, A., & Fabre, N. (2010). *Il Reve-eveille dirige in psicoterapia – via regia dell'immaginario* [The directed waking dream in psychotherapy – royal road to the imaginary]. Roma: Alpes.

Passerini, A., & Torlasco, S. (2011). *Psiconcologia e nuovi orizzonti nella terapia del cancro* [Psychoncology and new horizons in cancer therapy]. Roma: Alpes.

Passerini, A., & Vegetti, F. (2012). *Esperienza immaginativa: Counseling, pedagogia e psicoterapia* [Imaginative experience: Counselling, pedagogy and psychotherapy]. Roma: Alpes.

Pellerin, M., & Bres, M. (1994). La *Psychosynthese. Que sais-je?* [Psychosynthesis. What is it?]. Paris: Presses Universitaires de France.

Pepper, S. P. (1942). *World hypotheses: A study of evidence.* Berkeley: University of California Press.

Perry, C. (2008). Transference and countertransference. In P. Young-Eisendrath & T. Dawson (Eds.), *The Cambridge companion to Jung* (pp. 147–169). New York: Cambridge University Press.

Peters, E. (1978). *The magician, the witch, and the law.* Philadelphia: University of Pennsylvania Press.

Pietikäinen, P. (1999). *C. G. Jung and the psychology of symbolic forms.* Helsinki: Academia Scientiarum Fennica.

Pikes, N. (2005). *Dark voices: The genesis of Roy Hart theatre* (2nd edition). New Orleans, LA: Spring Journal Books.

Pivcevic, E. (1970). *Husserl and phenomenology.* London: Hutchnison university library.

Plaut, A. (1966). Reflections on not being able to imagine. *Journal of Analytical Psychology, 11*(2), 113–134.

Plateo-Zoja, S. (1978). *Analytical psychology and rêve eveillé dirigé* (Unpublished diploma thesis). C. G. Jung Institute, Zurich.

Politzer, G. (1994). *Critique of the foundations of psychology* (M. Apprey, Trans.). Pittsburgh, Pennsylvenia: Duquesne University Press. (Originally published in 1928).

Prinzhorn, H. (1922). *Artistry of the mentally ill.* New York: Springer-Verlag.

Progoff, I. (1975). *At a journal workshop.* New York: Dialogue House Library.

Rabassini, A. (1969). Comparative observations on methods of psychotherapy with mental imagery, the directed daydream of Desoille, the Rigo imaginative technique of psychotherapy and Jung's active imagination. *Rivista Sperimentale di Freniatria e Medicina Legale delle Alienazioni Mentali, 93*(6), 1360–1376.

Raff, J. (2000). *Jung and the alchemical imagination.* Berwick, Maine: Nicholas-Hays Inc.

Ragin, C. (1991). *Issues and alternatives in comparative social research.* Leiden: Brill.

Reddemann, L. (2008). *Psychodynamisch imaginative traumatherapie. PITT – Das Manual* [Psychodynamic imagery trauma therapy. PITT – The manual]. 5th ed. Stuttgart. Klett: Cotta.

Reik, T. (1948). *Listening with the third ear: The inner experience of a psychoanalyst.* New York: Grove Press.

Renaud, L. (1964). Application du R.E.D. à des amnesies retrogrades [Application of R.E.D. to retrograde amnesiacs]. *Bulletin de la Societé de recherché psychothérapiques de langue francaise, 2*(3), 9–11.

Reyher, J. (1977). Spontaneous visual imagery: Implications for psychoanalysis, psychopathology and psychotherapy. *Journal of Mental Imagery, 2*, 253–274.

Ribot, T. (1908). *Essai sur l'imagination créatrice* [Essay on the creative imagination]. Paris: Alcan.

Riceour, P. (1991). The function of fiction in shaping reality. In M. J. Valdes (Ed.), *A Ricoeur reader: Reflection and imagination* (pp. 448–462). Toronto: University of Toronto Press.

Riceour, P. (2004). *History, memory, forgetting*. Chicago, IL: University of Chicago Press.

Richet, C. (1922). *Traite de metapsychique*. Paris: Alcan.

Rigo, L. (1963). La psicoterapia con il rêve éveillé dirigé (Red) di poco spessore [Directed waking dream psychotherapy]. *Minerva Medicopsicologia, 4*, 3.

Rigo, L. (1965). La psicoterapia con il rêve éveillé dirigé [Directed waking dream psychotherapy]. Paris: Alcan. *Archivio di psicologia, neurologia, psiquiatria, 25*, 4–5.

Rigo, L. (1966). R.E.D. Diagnostico e Rorshcach contributo alla determinazione del fondo fantasmatico con mezzi psicodiagnostici [Diagnositc RED and Rorschach's contribution to the determination of the depth of fantasy with psychodiagnostic means]. Paris: Alcan. *Archivio di psicologia, neurologia, psiquiatria, 27*(4), V, 397–427.

Rigo, L. (1968). La tecnica immaginativa di analisi e ristrutturazione del profondo [The technique of imaginative analysis and restructuring in depth]. *Rivista Sperimentale di Freniatria e Medicina Legale delle Alienazioni Mentali., 93*, 6.

Rigo, L. (1970). L'lmagerie di gruppo negli adulti [Imagery in adult groups]. *Rivista Sperimentale di Freniatria e Medicina Legale delle Alienazioni Mentali, 94*, 5.

Rigo-Uberto, S. (1966–1967). *Il rêve éveillé dirigé in Francia ed in Italia* [The directed waking dream in France and Italy]. (Unpublished thesis). University of Turin, Italy.

Rocca, R. (1984). Diriger le rêve éveillé. [Directing the waking dream]. *Etudes Psychotherapiques, 57* (3), 217–228.

Rocca, R., & Stendoro, G. (2001). *L'immaginario – teatro delle nostre emozioni. Dal rêve- éveillé alla procedura immaginativa* [The imaginary – theatre of our emotions. From the waking dream to the imaginative experience]. Bologna: Clueb.

Rocca, R., & Stendoro, G. (2002). *Curare con l'immaginario* [Curing with the imaginary]. Roma: Armando.

Rocca, R., & Stendoro, G. (2005). *Psicosomatica – Una risposta dall'immaginario* [Psychosomatics – an answer from the imaginary]. Roma: Armando.

Rocca, R., & Villamarin, I. (2008). *El sueno despierto de Robert Desoille – un uso terapeutico de la imaginacion* [The waking dream of Robert Desoille – a therapeutic use of the imagination]. Quilmes, Argentina: Tiempo Sur.

Romanyshyn, R. (2007). *The wounded researcher: Research with soul in mind.* New Orleans: Spring Journal Books.

Rose, N. (1996). *Inventing ourselves: Psychology, power and personhood.* Cambridge: Cambridge University Press.

Rosenfeld, H. (1987). *Impasse and interpretation. Therapeutic and anti-therapeutic factors in the treatment of psychotic, borderline, and neurotic patients.* London: Tavistock Publications.

Rossi, M. A. (1990). Poetry as therapy: Self and world analysis. *Journal of Poetry Therapy, 3*, 167–171.

Roubineau, D. (1987). *Etude de l'évolution des concepts concernant le Reve-Eveille de Desoille à travers seize années d' "Etudes Psychothérapiques."* [A study of the development of concepts about the Waking-dream of Desoille over a seven year period of "Psychotherapeutic Studies"]. These de Doctorat en Médicine, Faculté de Médecine Pitie-Salpetriere, Université Pierre et Marie Curie (Paris 6).

Roudinesco, E. (1982). *La bataille de cent ans. Histoire de la psychoanalyse en France.* Vol. 1: 1885–1939 [The battle of hundred years. History of psychoanalysis in France. Volume 1: 1885–1939]. Paris: Ramsay.

Rousseau, J. J. (2013). *Emile.* Mineola, New York: Dover Publications. (Originally published in 1911).

Rowland, S. (2013). Reading Jung for magic: "Active Imagination" for/as "Close reading". In J. Kirsch & M. Stein (Eds.), *How and why we still read Jung* (pp. 86–105). New York: Routledge.

Rust, M. J., & Totton, N. (2012). *Vital Signs: Psychological responses to ecological crisis.* London: Karnac Books.

Sabini, M. (2002). *The earth has a soul: Jung on nature, technology and modern life.* Berkeley, CA: North Atlantic Books.

Safran, J. D. (2012). *Psychoanalysis and psychoanalytic therapies.* Washington, DC: American Psychological Association.

Safran, J. D., & Muran, C. J. (2000). *Negotiating the therapeutic alliance: A relational treatment guide.* New York: The Guilford Press.

Salman, S. (2010). Peregrinations of active imagination – The elusive quintessence in the postmodern labyrinth. In M. Stein (Ed.), *Jungian psychoanalysis: Working in the spirit of C. G. Jung* (pp. 118–133). La Salle, IL: Open Court.

Sapir, E. (1921). *Language: An introduction to the study of speech.* New York: Harcourt, Brace and Company.

Samuels, A. (1985a). *Jung and the post-Jungians.* London: Routledge & Kegan Paul.

Samuels, A. (1985b). Counter-transference, the *'Mundus Imaginalis'* and the Research project. *Journal of Analytical Psychology, 30,* 47–71.

Samuels, A. (1989a). *The plural psyche.* London: Routledge.

Samuels, A. (1989b). Analysis and pluralism: The politics of the psyche. *The Journal of Analytical Psychology, 34,* 33–51.

Samuels, A. (1994). Jung and anti-semitism. *Jewish Quarterly, 40*(5), 59–63.

Samuels, A. (2006). Transference/countertransference. In R. K. Papadopoulos (Ed.), *The handbook of Jungian psychology: Theory, practice and applications* (pp. 177–195). New York: Routledge.

Samuels, A. (2008). New developments in the post-Jungian field. In P. Young-Eisendrath & T. Dawson (Eds.), *The Cambridge companion to Jung* (2nd ed., pp. 1–15). New York: Cambridge University Press.

Samuels, A. (2014). Shadows of the therapy relationship. In D. Loewenthal & A. Samuels (Eds.), *Relational psychotherapy, psychoanalysis and counselling* (pp. 184–192). London and New York: Routledge.

Samuels, A. (2015). *Passions, persons, psychotherapy, politics. The selected writings of Andrew Samuels.* London and New York: Routledge.

Sapir, E. (1921). *Language: An introduction to the study of speech.* New York: Harcourt, Brace.

Sapir, M. (1975). *La relaxation à inductions variables* [Relaxation with different inductions]. Grenoble: La pensée sauvage.

Sassenfeld, A. (2007). Del cuerpo individual a un cuerpo relacional: Dimensión somática, interacción y cambio en psicoterapia [From the individual body towards a relational body: Somatic dimension, interaction, and change in psychotherapy]. *Gaceta de Psiquiatría Universitaria*, *3*(2), 177–188.

Savage, J. A. (2011). Trust and betrayal: Four women under Jung's shadow. In S. Wirth, I. Meier, J. Hill (Eds.), *Trust & Betrayal: Dawnings of Consciousness, Jungian Odyssey Series*, Volume 3, (pp. 101–116). New Orleans: Spring Journal Publications.

Schafer, R. (1980). Narration in the psychoanalytic dialogue: Psychoanalytic theories as narratives. *Critical Inquiry*, *7*(1), 29–53.

Schaverien, J. (1982, Sept). Transference as an aspect of art therapy. *Inscape*, 10–16.

Schaverien, J. (1987). The scapegoat and the talisman. Transference in art therapy. In T. Dalley, T., C. Case & J. Schaverien (Eds.), *Images of art therapy*. London and New York: Routledge.

Schaverien, J. (1999). *The revealing image: Analytical art psychotherapy in theory and practice*. London and New York: Jessica Kingsley. (Originally published in 1991).

Schaverien, J. (2000). The triangular relationship and the aesthetic countertransference in analytical art psychotherapy. In A. Gilroy & G. McNeilly (Eds.), *The changing shape of art therapy: New developments in theory and practise* (pp. 55–83). London: Jessica Kingsley Publisher.

Schaverien, J. (2005a). Art and active imagination: Further reflections on transference and the image. *The International Journal of Art Therapy: Inscape*, *10*(2), 39–52.

Schaverien, J. (2005b). Art dreams and active imagination: A post-Jungian approach to transference and the image. *Journal of Analytical Psychology*, *50*(2), 127–153.

Schaverien, J. (2007). Countertransference as active imagination: Imaginative experiences of the analyst. *Journal of Analytical Psychology*, *52*, 413–431.

Schaverien, J. (2008). Active imagination and countertransference enchantment: Space and time within the analytic frame. In L. Huskinson (Ed.), *Dreaming the myth onwards: New directions in Jungian therapy and thought* (pp. 122–131). New York: Routledge.

Schaverien, J., & Case, C. (2007). *Supervision in art psychotherapy: A theoretical and practical handbook*. Hove: Routledge.

Schnetzler, J. P. (1967). Traitement d'un cas de psychose maniac-depressive par le R.E.D. [Treatment of a case of a psychotic manic-depressive with R.E.D.]. *Bulletin de la Societe de Recherché Psychotherapiques de Langue Francaise*, *5*(1), 25–29.

Schorr, J. E. (1972). *Psycho-imagination therapy. The integration of phenomenology and imagination*. New York: Intercontinental Medical Book Corporation.

Schultz, J. H. (1958). *Le training autogene. Methode de relaxation par auto-décontraction concentrative* [Autogenic training. A method of relaxation with concentrative auto-decontraction]. Paris: Presses Universitaries de France. (Originally published in 1932).

Schwartz-Salant, N. (1986). On the subtle body concept in clinical practice. In N. Schwartz-Salant & M. Stein (Eds.), *The body in analysis*. Wilmette: Chiron Publications.

Schwartz-Salant, N. (1988). Archetypal foundations of projective identification. *Journal of Analytical Psychology*, *33*, 39–64.

Schwartz-Salant, N. (1989). *The borderline personality: Vision and healing.* Wilmette, IL: Chiron Publications.

Schwartz-Salant, N. (1995). On the interactive field as the analytic object. In M. Stein (Ed.), *The interactive field in analysis* (pp. 1–36). Wilmette: Chiron.

Schwartz-Salant, N. (1998). *The mystery of human relationships: Alchemy and the transformation of the self.* London and New York: Routledge.

Schwartz-Salant, N. (2010). The mark of one who has seen chaos. A review of C. G. Jung's Red Book. *Quadrant,* xxxx(2), 11–38.

Segal, H. (1952). A psychoanalytical approach to aesthetics. *International Journal of Psychoanalysis, 33,* 196–207.

Segal, S. J., & Glickman, M. (1967). Relaxation and the Perky effect: The influence of body position and judgements of imagery. *American Journal of Psychology, 80*(2), 257–262.

Sedgwick, D. (1994). *The wounded healer: Countertransference from a Jungian perspective.* New York: Routledge.

Sedgwick, D. (2001). *Introduction to Jungian psychotherapy: The therapeutic relationship.* New York: Routledge.

Serina, F. (2013). 'La structure de l'âme' de C. G. Jung (Genève, Juin 1928) ["The structure of the soul" of C. G. Jung]. *Revue de Psychologie Analytique, 1,* 177–196.

Serina, F. (2018). C, G. Jung's encounter with the French Readers. The Paris lecture May (1934). *Phanes - Journal for Jung History, 1,* 112–137.

Serrano, P. G. (1999). Catábasis y resurrección [Katabasis and resurrection]. *Espacio, Tiempo y Forma, Serie II: Historia Antigua, 12,* 129–179.

Shamdasani, S. (1995). Memories, dreams, *omissions. Spring: Journal of Archetype and Culture, 57,* 115–137.

Shamdasani, S. (2003/2004). *Jung and the making of modern psychology.* Cambridge: Cambridge University Press.

Shamdasani, S. (2005). *Jung stripped bare by his biographers.* Even, London and New York: Karnac Books.

Shamdasani, S. (2009). Introduction. *The Red Book: Liber Novus* (pp. 193–224). New York: Norton.

Shamdasani, S. (2012a). *C. G. Jung: A biography in books.* New York and London: W. W. Norton & Company.

Shamdasani, S. (2012b). After Liber Novus. *Journal of Analytical Psychology, 57,* 364–377.

Shantz, D. E. (2013). *An introduction to German Pietism.* Baltimore: John Hopkins.

Shaw, B. G. (1904). *Man and superman: A comedy and a philosophy.* New York: Brentano's.

Sheikh, A. A., & Jordan, C. S. (1983). Clinical uses of mental imagery. In A. A. Sheikh (Ed.), *Imagery, current theory, research, and application* (pp. 391–435). New York: John Wiley & Sons.

Silberer, H. (1909). Bericht über eine Methode, gewisse symbolische Halluzinations-Erscheinungen hervorzurufen und zu beobachten [Report on a method to elicit certain observable symbolic hallucinatory phenomena]. *Jahrbuch für psychoanalytische und psychopathologische Forschungen, 2,* 541–622.

Silver, R. (2001). *Art as language: Access to emotions and cognitive skills through drawings.* London: Brunner-Routledge.

Simon, R. (1995). *The symbolism of style*. London: Routledge.

Simpson, H. M., & Paivio, A. (1966). Changes in pupil size during an imagery task. *Psycho-nomic Science, 13*, 293–294.

Simmonton, O. C., Matthews-Simmonton, S., & Creighton, J. L. (1978). *Getting well again*. New York: Bantam Books.

Singer, J. L., & Antrobus, J. S. (1972). Daydreaming, imaginal processes, and personality: A normative study. In P. W. Sheehan (Ed.), *The nature and function of imagery* (pp. 175–202). New York: Academic Press.

Singer, J. (1972). *Boundaries of the soul: The practice of Jung's psychology*. Garden City, NY: Anchor Books.

Sivadon, P. (1967). Hommage à Monsieur Robert Desoille. [Homage to Mr. Robert Desoille]. *Bulletin de la Société de Recherché Psychothérapiques de Langue Francaise, V, 1*, Mars, 3–4.

Skaar, P. (2002). The goal as process: Music and the search for self. *Journal of Analytical Psychology, 47*, 629–638.

Slattery, P. D. (2011). Thirteen ways of looking at the Red Book: C. G. Jung's Divine Comedy. *Jung Journal: Culture & Psyche, 5*(3), 128–144.

Smelser, N. (1976). *Comparative methods in the social sciences*. Englewood Cliffs, NJ: Prentice Hall.

Soja, E. (1989). *Postmodern human geographies. The reassertion of space in critical social theory*. London: Verso.

Soja, E. (1996). *Thirdspace. A journey into Los Angeles and other real-and-imagined places*. Oxford: Blackwell.

Sokolov, L. (1987). Vocal improvisation therapy. In K. Bruscia (Ed.), *Improvisational models of music therapy* (pp. 353–359). University Park, IL: Barcelona Publishers.

Solie, P. (1971, Juillet-Octobre). Psychologie analytique et imagerie mentale [Analytical psychology and mental imagery]. *Psychotherapies: Revue de l'Arbre Vert, 3*, 11–13.

Sorge, G. (2009). Love as Devotion. Olga Fröbe-Kapteyn's relationship with Eranos and Jungian Psychology. In *Eranos-Yearbook–Annale di Eranos 70*, 2009–2010–2011, Love on a Fragile Thread – L'amore sul filo della fragilità, hg. von F. Merlini, L. E. Sullivan, R. Bernardini und K. Olson, Daimon Verlag, Einsiedeln 2012, S. 388–434.

Smelser, N. (1976). *Comparative methods in the social sciences*. Engelwood Cliffs, NJ: Prentice Hall.

Smith, M. (1978). *Jesus the magician*. San Francisco, CA: Harper & Row.

Smucker, M. R. (1997). Post-traumatic stress disorder. In R. L. Leahy (Ed.), *Practicing cognitive therapy: A guide to interventions* (pp. 193–220). Northvale, NJ: Jason Aronson.

Stein, M. (2006). Individuation. In R. K. Papadopoulos (Ed.), *The handbook of Jungian psychology: Theory, practice and applications* (pp. 196–214). New York: Routledge.

Stein, M. (2012). How to read *The Red Book* and why. *Journal of Analytical Psychology, 57*, 280–298.

Stein, M., & Brutsche, P. (2009). *Active imagination & the use of images in Jungian analysis*. The Asheville Jung Center. (Producer). [DVD] AJC Seminar #4.

Stephani, L. Stephens. (2019). *C. G. Jung and the dead: Visions, active imagination and the unconscious terrain*. London: Routledge.

Stewart, L. (1987). Affect and archetype in analysis. In N. Schwartz-Salant & M. Stein (Eds.), *Archetypal processes in psychotherapy*, (pp. 131–162). Wilmette III: Chiron Publications.

Stoeffler, F. E. (1965). *The rise of evangelical pietism.* Lieden: E. J. Brill.

Storr, A. (1992). *Music and the mind.* London: Harpercollins.

Stricker, G., & Gold, J. R. (1996). Psychotherapy integration: An assimilative, psychodynamic approach. *Clinical Psychology: Science and Practice, 3,* 47–58.

Strupp, H. H., & Binder, J. L. (1984). *Psychotherapy in a new key.* New York: Basic Books.

Suler, J. R. (2004). The online disinhibition effect. *Cyber Psychology and Behavior, 7,* 321–326.

Swan, W. (2007). *C. G. Jung and active imagination.* Germany: VDM Verlag.

Taylor, C. (1989). *Sources of the self.* Cambridge: Cambridge University Press.

Tchou, C. (Ed.). (1964). Hervey de Saint-Denys, *Les Rêves et les Moyens de les Diriger.* [Dream and the means to direct them]. Paris: Bibliothèque du Merveilleux. (Originally published in 1867).

Telle, J. (Ed.). (1992). *Rosarium philosophorum.: Ein alchememisches florilegium des spatmittelalters.* 2 Vols. Weinheim: VCH.

Teo, T. (2005). *The critique of psychology: From Kant to postcolonial theory.* New York: Springer.

Ternoy, M. (1997). *Rorschach, rêve eveillé dirigé et expression grapho-picturale dans l'etude phenomeno-structurale des hallucinations* [Rorschach, directed waking dream and the graphical-pictorial expression in the phenomenological-structural study of hallucinations]. Mikrofiche: Ausg.

Thackery, S. (2014). Manifesting the vision: C. G. Jung's paintings for the Red Book. In T. Kirsch & G. Hogenson (Eds.), *The Red Book: Reflections on C. G. Jung's Liber Novus* (pp. 67–80). New York: Routledge.

Thibaudier, V. (2011). *100% Jung.* Paris: Éditions Eyrolles.

Thirion-Henault, M. (1973). Dynamique de l'imaginaire dans le RED de Desoille [They dynamic of the imaginary in the RED of Desoille]. *Bulletin de zPsychologie, 27,* 5–9.

Thomas, V. (2016). *Using mental imagery in counselling and psychotherapy: A guide to more inclusive theory and practice.* London and New York: Routledge.

Tibaldi, M. (2004). Psicoterapia analitica ed EMDR: un avvicinamento possibile? [Analytic psychotherapy and EMDR: A possible coming together?]. *Studi Junghiani, 20,* Luglio-Dicembre, 127–144.

Tilly, M. (1956/1977). The therapy of music. In McGuire & Hull (Eds.), *C. G. Jung Speaking* (pp. 273–275). Princeton, NJ: Princeton University Press.

Todorov, T. (1975). *The fantastic: A structural approach to a literary genre.* Ithaca, NY: Cornell University Press.

Tosh, J. (1984). *The pursuit of history: Aims, methods and new directions in the study of modern history.* London: Longman.

Totton, N. (2003). *Body psychotherapy: An introduction.* Maidenhead: Open University Press.

Turner, E., & Turner, V. (1978). *Image and pilgrimage in Christian culture. Anthropological perspectives.* New York: Columbia University Press.

Turner, B. (2005). *The handbook of sandplay therapy.* Cloverdale, CA: Tenemos Press.

Ulanov, B. A. (2010). God climbs down to morality – Jung in his Red Book. *Quadrant*, xxxx(2), 61–78.

Valtorta, F., & Passerini, A. (2015). *Resilienza ed esperienza immaginativa: Come utilizzare l'immaginario per affrontare trauma, stress, difficolta'e promuovere la crescita personale* [Reslience and imaginative experience: How to utilise the imagination to treat trauma, stress and difficulties and how to promote personal development]. Rome: Alpes.

van der Kolk, B. (2014). *The body knows the score. Brain, mind and body in the healing of trauma.* New York: Viking Press.

van Loben Sels, R. (2003). *A dream in the world: Poetics of soul in two women, modern and medieval.* New York: Brunner-Routledge.

Velletri, T. (2015). *Mircea Eliade and C. G. Jung: A comparative study* (Unpublished doctoral thesis). University of Essex - Centre for Psychoanalytic Studies, UK.

Villamarin, I. (1995). El sueno despierto acompanante [The guided waking dream]. *Revista Sueno despierto, 3.* Bueonos Aires.

Virel, A. (1965). *Histoire de notre image.* [A history of our image]. Geneve: Mont-Blanc.

Virel, A., & Fretigny, R. (1968). *L'imagerie Mentale: introduction a l'onirotherapie.* [mental imagery: An introduction to oneirotherapy]. Geneve: Mont-Blanc.

Virel, A. (1970–1971). Approches psychophysiologiques de l'imagerie mentale. [Psychophysiological approaches of mental imagery]. *Bulletin de psychologie, 291,* XXIV, 9–11.

Virel, A. (1977). *Vocabulaire des psychotherapies.* Paris: Fayard.

Vittoz, R. (1937). *Traitement des psychonevroses par le re-education du controle cerebral* [Treatment of psychoneurosis through the re-education and cerebral control]. Paris: Bailliere. (Originally published in 1911).

van Engen, J. H. (1988). *Devotio moderna: Basic writings.* Mahwah, NJ: Paulist Press.

van Loben Sels, R. (2003). *A dream in the world: Poetics of soul in two women, modern and medieval.* New York: Brunner-Routledge.

Virshup, E. (1978). *Right-brained people in a left-brained world.* Los Angeles: Guild of Tutors Press.

von Franz, M. L., & Hillman, J. (1971). *Jung's typology.* New York: Spring Publications.

von Franz, M. L. (1974). *Shadow and evil in fairy tales.* Zurich: Spring.

von Franz, M. L. (1980). On active imagination. In I. F. Baker (Ed.), *Methods of treatment in analytical psychology – V11 International congress of the international association for analytical psychology* (pp. 88–99). Fellbach: Bonz.

von Franz, M. L. (1980). On active imagination. In *Inward Journey: Art as therapy* (pp. 125–133). La Salle, IL and London: Open Court, 1983.

von Franz, M. L. (1993). *Psychotherapy.* Boston: Shambala.

Wachtel, P. L. (2008). *Relational theory and the practice of psychotherapy.* New York: Guilford Press.

Warren, J. (1999). *History and the historians.* London: Hodder & Stoughton.

Watkins. M. (1976). *Waking dreams.* New York: Harper Colophon Books.

Watkins, H. (2011). *Metaphors of depth in German musical thought: From E.T.A. Hoffmann Arnold Shoenberg.* Cambridge: Cambridge University Press.

Weaver, R. (1991). *The old wise woman: A study of active imagination.* Boston: Shambala. (Originally published in 1973).

Wehr, G. (1987). *Jung: A biography*. Boston: Shambala Publications.

Weiner, D. (1999). *Beyond talk therapy: Using movement and expressive techniques in clinical practice*. Washington, DC: American Psychological Association.

Weiner, J. (2009). *The therapeutic relationship – transference, countertransference and the making of meaning*. College Station: Texas A & M University Press.

Wellisch, E. (1950). Active imagination during the use of the Rorschach method. *The British Journal of Psychiatry, 96*(403), 476–483.

White, M., & Epson, D. (1990). *Narrative means to therapeutic ends*. New York: W. W. Norton & Co.

Williams, T. (1945). *The glass menagerie*. New York: Random House.

Winnicott, D. W. (1974). The capacity to be alone. In D. W. Winnicott, *The maturational processes and the facilitating environment: Studies in the theory of emotional development* (pp. 29–36). New York: International Universities Press, Inc. (Originally published in 1958).

Winnicott, D. W. (1960). The theory of the parent-infant relationship. In D. W. Winnicott (Ed.), *The maturational processes and the facilitating environment* (pp. 233–253). Madison, CT: International Universities Press.

White, M., & Epston, D. (1990). *Narrative means to therapeutic ends*. New York: W. W. Norton.

Whitehouse, M. (1979). C. G. Jung and dance therapy. In P. Lewis Bernstein (Ed.), *Eight theoretical approaches in dance-movement therapy* (pp. 51–70). Dubuque: Kendall/Hunt.

Whitmont, C. E., & Pereira, B. S. (1989). *Dreams, a portal to the source*. London: Routledge.

Wojtkowski, S. (2009). Jung's art complex. *Art & Psyche Online Journal*, (3). (Retrieved from: https://aras.org/newsletter/newsletter09-03.htm)

Wolff, T. (1956). *Structural forms of the feminine psyche* (P. Watzlawik, Trans.). Zurich: Privately printed for the C.G, Jung Institute.

Wood, M. (1984). The child and art therapy: A psychodynamic viewpoint. In T. Dalley (Ed.), *Art as therapy* (pp. 62–81). London: Tavistock.

Wood, C. (1990). The triangular relationship (1): The beginnings and the endings of art therapy. *Inscape: Journal of Art Therapy*, Winter, 7–13.

Woodman, M. (1980). *The Owl was a baker's daughter: Obesity, anorexia nervosa, and the repressed feminine*. Toronto: Inner City Books.

Woodman, M. (1982). *Addiction to Perfection*. New York: Basic Books.

Wunenburger, J. J. (1991). *L'imaginaire*, Que sais-je? [The imaginary, what is it?]. Paris: Presses Universitaires de France.

Wyman-McGinty, W. (1998). The body in analysis: Authentic movement and witnessing in analytic practice. *Journal of Analytical Psychology, 43*(2), 239–260.

Young, R. J. C. (1995). *Colonial desire: Hybridity in theory, culture and race*. London and New York: Routledge.

Zalewski, E. F. (1971). *Rapports entre le rêve éveillé dirigé de Robert Desoille et la théorie de C. G. Jung* [The relationship between the directed waking dream of Robert Desoille and the theory of C. G. Jung]. (Thèse inédite), Universite de Grenoble, France.

Zanetti, M. A., Passerini, A., & De Palma, M. (2010). *Strategie a confronto nell'integrazione delle culture diverse* [Strategies for an integration of different cultures]. Roma: Alpes.

Biographical details of Robert Desoille

Robert Emile Charles Desoille was born at no. 3, Rue de Lorraine in Besancon, Doubs in the Franche Comté region of France on May 29, 1890. His father was named Emile Ildefonse. The latter was born on February 6, 1851 at 32 Rue Grenata in Paris and was the son of Isidore Joseph and Narcisse Sophie Ledru. Desoille's father married Fanny Marie Louise Loonen (Desoille's mother) on June 18, 1888. Fanny Marie Louise Loonen was born in Paris on July 30, 1865. She did not work and resided at Rue de Marignan, Paris. She was the daughter of Ferdinand Hubert Adrien Loonen (1824–1884) and Luise Justine Demont-Rond (1829–1908).

Emile Ildefonse served in the military for 40 years and reached the rank of a military general. He died on April 9, aged 63, and was given a military funeral. Robert was 24 when he lost his father. Emile Ildefonse and Fanny had two children, Robert and Henri. Henri, the second child, was born on December 11, 1900 and was given the names of Marie, Felix and Emile. He became a professor of medicine at the Faculty of Medicine in Paris. Henri married Paule Leonie Desoille Merlhes. He lived at no. 47, Boulevard Garibaldi, Paris. He was taken as prisoner in Mounthausen-Gusen in Austria during the Second World War. Luckily he survived the concentration camp. He died later in 1974.

Robert studied engineering at the University of Lille and graduated in 1911. He wanted to continue to study physiological psychology at the Sorbonne University; however, because of the First World War he had to abandon this project. He took part in this war and was wounded. He was decorated with the military cross and was awarded the French Legion of honour. Robert later worked as an engineer until 1953 with *Electricité et du Gaz de France*. During the Second World War, he was stationed at Cery, France and formed part of the Resistance.

Robert married twice. His first wife was Lucie Madeleine Marguerite Marie Bigeard from Pellouailles. The couple married on June 29, 1920. When Lucie died, Robert re-married Mireille Paule Leona d'Ambrosio, from Nice, on October 14, 1950 (the date 1940 on the marriage certificate must be wrong, since Lucie, his first wife, was still alive – the correct date features as a later addition on the side of Desoille's birth certificate). Robert Desoille never had children. The only niece he had was Mme. Monique Pellerin. She also became a psychotherapist. Desoille first lived at 9, Rue Falguiere, Paris, Xve in the Montparnasse quarter in Paris. Then he moved later in his life to no. 4. Rue Chambiges, Paris.

Robert died on October 10, 1966, in his home, at Rue Chambiges. He is buried at the famous *Père Lachaise* cemetery in Paris, in the family tomb which belonged to his mother's family at the 24th division. The epitaph reads: Robert Desoille 1890–1966 – PRIEZ POUR EUX/PRAY FOR THEM.

Index